Plato's Press

CHICAGO, ILLINOIS



THE LIBRARY
OF Congress HAS
CATALOGUED THIS TEXT AS FOLLOWS
Registration: XXX

Volume 2

# BIOETHICS
## Program Director's
# HANDBOOK
## Leading with Integrity and Compassion

Description: Electronic File (eService)
Copyright: Jeffrey Wallace Bulger
Date of Creation: 8/15/2024
Authorship: Jeffrey Wallace Bulger
Rights and Permissions: Jeffrey Wallace Bulger

ISBN 978-1-62252-031-2
9 781622 520312

# Volume 2 BIOETHICS Program Director's HANDBOOK

## Leading with Integrity and Compassion

---

## Book Description

---

**Volume 2 of the Healthcare Ethics Handbook Series**

In today's healthcare landscape, ethical leadership is essential for fostering collaboration and integrity. *Volume 2 — Bioethics Program Director's Handbook: Leading with Integrity and Compassion*, the second volume in the *Healthcare Ethics Handbook Series*, equips bioethics program directors with the expertise and tools necessary for effective leadership. Building on the frameworks introduced in Volume 1, this volume offers strategic insights into managing bioethics programs, shaping policies, and promoting a culture of ethical awareness across healthcare institutions.

**Key Features**:

- **Understanding the Role of a Bioethics Program Director**: Learn key responsibilities and leadership skills.
- **Core Responsibilities**: Conduct ethics consultations, develop policies, and implement preventive strategies.
- **Enhancing Communication and Education**: Master communication techniques and ethics education, including workshops and simulations.
- **Leveraging Technology for Bioethics**: Integrate ethics into electronic health records (EHR) and digital tools.

- **Continuous Improvement and Professional Development**: Methods for refining consultations and encouraging growth.
- **Leading with Integrity and Compassion**: Inspire ethical leadership and high standards.
- **Practical Tools and Resources**: Templates, checklists, and policy guidelines for ethical education.
- **Real-World Case Studies**: Analyze complex ethical dilemmas to enhance decision-making skills.
- **Review Questions and Further Readings**: Reinforce understanding with review questions and additional readings.

**About the Series:**

The *Healthcare Ethics Handbook Series* is a three-volume resource for healthcare professionals navigating ethical challenges. Volume 1 covers ethical decision-making and clinical consultation, Volume 2 focuses on bioethics leadership and policy development, and Volume 3 addresses 60 clinical ethics topics. The series is grounded in bioethical principles, equipping readers for ethical leadership.

**About the Author:**

Dr. Jeffrey W. Bulger brings both academic and practical expertise to medical ethics. His recent book, *Bioethics: Passing the Boards, Providing Patient Care, and Beyond*, published by Oxford University Press, reflects his dedication to guiding healthcare professionals through ethical challenges.

***

# Table of Contents

**Part I: Understanding the Role of a Bioethics Program Director .......1**

**Chapter 1: Introduction to Bioethics Program Leadership ........................1**

Defining Bioethics ........................................................................1

Bioethical Principles ......................................................................2

The Role of the Bioethics Program Director .............................................4

Integrating Ethical Principles in Leadership..............................................6

Key Skills and Qualities for Effective Leadership ......................................6

1.1 Leadership Self-Assessment Tool.......................................................9

1.2 Ethical Dilemma Case Documentation Form ......................................14

1.3 Ethics Program Development Checklist .............................................16

1.4 Stakeholder Engagement Template....................................................18

1.5 Program Director's Monthly Report Template ....................................20

Further Readings and References ..........................................................22

**Chapter 2: Building a Strong Foundation ..................................................25**

Integrating Bioethics with Organizational Strategy..................................25

Evaluating and Communicating the Impact of Bioethics Initiatives .........26

Integrating Bioethics into All Organizational Levels ...............................27

Establishing and Leading the Bioethics Committee .................................27

Creating a Culture of Ethical Sensitivity and Collaboration .....................28

Implementing Ethical Guidelines and Protocols........................................29

2.1 Strategic Alignment Checklist ..........................................................32

2.2 Bioethics Committee Member Selection Form...................................34

2.3 Bioethics Committee Meeting Agenda Template ...............................36

2.4 Ethical Sensitivity and Collaboration Action Plan..............................38

Further Readings and References .........................................................40

**Chapter 3: Developing a Mission, Vision and Values Statement.............43**

The Role of Mission, Vision, and Values Statements ...............................43

Developing the Mission Statement.........................................................44

Case Study: Crafting a Mission Statement ..............................................45

Crafting a Vision Statement...................................................................46

Case Study: Developing a Vision Statement ...........................................48

Involving Stakeholders .........................................................................48

Regular Review and Adaptation ............................................................49

Practical Steps for Alignment with Mission and Vision Statements..........49

Case Study: Aligning with Mission and Vision .......................................50

Integrating TAC with SOAP: Enhancing Ethical Documentation.............51

Case Study: Integrating TAC with SOAP...............................................53

Setting Short-term and Long-term Goals.................................................54

Short-Term Goals Examples: .................................................................54

Long-Term Goals Examples: .................................................................56

Case Study: Setting Goals.....................................................................58

Resource Considerations....58
Developing the Values Statement....61
Values Statement:....62
Communicating the Mission, Vision, and Values to Stakeholders....62
3.1 Mission Statement Development Template....66
3.2 Vision Statement Development Template....68
3.3 Values Statement Development Template....70
3.4 Communication Plan Template....72
Further Readings and References....74

**Review Questions....77**

**Part II: Core Responsibilities of a Bioethics Program Director....81**

**Chapter 4: Conducting Healthcare Ethics Consultations....81**

Overview of Healthcare Ethics Consultations....81
Establishing Clear Protocols....82
Addressing Systemic Issues....83
Interprofessional Collaboration....83
Case Study 1: End-of-Life Decision-Making in a Interprofessional Context 84
Training and Education....85
Monitoring and Evaluation....85
Consultation Process:....86
Integrating Ethics Consultations into Quality Improvement....86
Encouraging Peer Support and Mentoring....87
4.1 Structured Process for Ethics Consultations....89
— I. Initiating an Ethics Consultation....89
— II. Gathering Information....89
— III. Conducting the Consultation....90
— IV. Providing Support....90
— V. Monitoring and Evaluation....91
— VI. Addressing Systemic Issues....91
4.2 TAC Methodology & SOAP Documentation....92
4.3 SOAP Notes....97
— (S) Subjective....97
— (O) Objective....98
— (A) Assessment....99
— (P) Plan....99
4.4 SOAP Notes—Cue Card....101
4.5 Post-Consultation Survey....102
4.6 Follow-Up Interview....108
4.7 Feedback Forms....112
Further Readings and References....116

**Chapter 5: Policy Development and Organizational Ethics....119**

Developing and Reviewing Policies....119
Key Principles in Policy Development:....119
Steps for Policy Development....120
Ensuring Compliance with Regulatory Standards and Ethical Norms:...121

Case Study: Informed Consent Policy Development ..... 122
5.1/15.1 Policy Development Template ..... 125
5.2 Policy Development, Review, and Revision Checklist ..... 128
5.3 Policy Implementation and Communication ..... 131
5.4 Informed Consent Policy Template ..... 133
5.5 Policy Feedback Form ..... 136
Further Readings and References ..... 138

**Chapter 6: Preventive Ethics ..... 141**
Importance of Preventive Ethics ..... 141
Core Principles in Preventive Ethics: ..... 141
Implementing Preventive Ethics Strategies: ..... 142
Fostering a Culture of Ethical Vigilance: ..... 143
Addressing Systemic Issues ..... 144
Monitoring and Evaluation ..... 145
6.1 Ethics Rounds Discussion Template ..... 147
6.2 Ethical Risk Assessment Form ..... 149
6.3 Incident Reporting Form for Ethical Concerns ..... 151
6.4 Preventive Ethics Activity Log ..... 153
6.5 Ethics Audit Checklist ..... 155
Further Readings and References ..... 157

**Review Questions ..... 159**

**Part III: Enhancing Communication and Education ..... 163**

**Chapter 7: Effective Communication in Ethics Consultation ..... 163**
Techniques for Active Listening and Empathetic Engagement ..... 163
Empathetic Engagement ..... 164
Training and Development ..... 164
Mediating Conflicts and Facilitating Consensus ..... 165
Key Mediation Techniques ..... 165
Training in Mediation Skills ..... 166
Ensuring Clear and Balanced Ethical Advice ..... 166
Documentation and Protocols ..... 167
Promoting a Culture of Ethical Awareness ..... 168
7.1 Active Listening and Empathetic Engagement Training Worksheet . 170
7.2 Mediation and Conflict Resolution Protocol ..... 172
7.3 Ethics Consultation Summary Template ..... 174
7.4 Reflective Practice and Peer Feedback Form ..... 176
7.5 Communication Skills Workshop Evaluation Form ..... 178
Further Readings and References ..... 180

**Chapter 8: Designing and Delivering Ethics Education Programs ..... 183**
Creating Engaging and Effective Training Sessions ..... 183
Tailoring Content to the Audience ..... 184
Ongoing Learning and Development ..... 185
Using Interactive Workshops, Case Studies, and Simulations ..... 185
Incorporating Technology in Interactive Education ..... 186
Evaluating and Improving Education Programs ..... 186
Incorporating Best Practices and Emerging Trends ..... 187

Conducting Research to Measure Impact ........ 187
8.1 Training Session Planning Template ........ 189
8.2 Participant Feedback Form for Training Sessions ........ 191
8.3 Case Study Analysis Worksheet ........ 193
8.4 Simulation Scenario Template ........ 195
8.5 Ethics Education Program Evaluation Form ........ 197
Further Readings and References ........ 199
**Chapter 9: Outreach and Professional Engagement ........ 201**
Organizing Workshops, Seminars, and Conferences: ........ 201
Collaborating with Other Bioethics Leaders ........ 202
Promoting the Visibility and Impact of the Bioethics Program ........ 202
Educating the General Public ........ 203
Participating in Policy Discussions and Advocacy ........ 204
Engaging with Local, State, National, and International Communities ..204
Building Networks and Collaborations ........ 206
Engaging in Joint Research and Training Programs ........ 206
Promoting Visibility and Credibility ........ 207
9.1 Outreach and Professional Engagement Planning Template ........ 209
9.2 Participant Feedback Form for Outreach Events ........ 211
9.3 Networking and Collaboration Log ........ 213
9.4 Outreach Program Evaluation Template ........ 214
9.5 Policy Advocacy Planning Template ........ 216
Further Readings and References ........ 218
**Review Questions ........ 221**
**Part IV: Leveraging Technology for Bioethics ........ 225**
**Chapter 10: Integrating Ethics into Electronic Health Records (EHR)...225**
Utilizing the EHR System for Ethical Documentation ........ 225
Promoting the Use of EHR for Ethical Decision-Making ........ 226
Best Practices for Using SOAP Notes in Ethics Consultation ........ 227
Integrating SOAP Notes Across Clinical Practice ........ 228
Ensuring Transparency and Accountability in EHR ........ 228
Implementing Regular Audits and Reviews ........ 229
Leveraging Technology for Enhanced Transparency ........ 229
10.1 EHR Ethical Documentation Customization Request Form ........ 231
10.2 SOAP Notes EHR Integration ........ 233
10.3 EHR Ethical Documentation Audit Checklist ........ 235
10.4 EHR Ethical Documentation Training Agenda ........ 237
Further Readings and References ........ 239
**Chapter 11: Using Technology to Enhance Ethics Programs ........ 241**
Implementing Digital Tools for Ethics Rounds and Training ........ 241
Promoting Digital Tool Usage ........ 242
Enhancing Collaboration with Digital Tools ........ 242
Leveraging Data Analytics for Ethics Quality Improvement ........ 243
Promoting Data-Driven Ethics Quality Improvement ........ 244
Ensuring Accessibility and User-Friendliness ........ 244
Exploring Future Trends in Bioethics Technology ........ 245

Fostering a Culture of Innovation and Continuous Improvement ........... 245
Addressing Ethical Implications of Emerging Technologies ........... 246
11.1 Digital Tools Implementation Plan ........... 248
11.2 Data Analytics Metrics and Dashboard Development Guide ........... 250
11.3 Emerging Technology Exploration Template ........... 252
Further Readings and References ........... 254

**Review Questions ........... 257**

**Part V: Continuous Improvement and Professional Development. 261**

**Chapter 12: Analyzing and Improving Consultation Methods ........... 261**
Regularly Reviewing and Evaluating Processes ........... 261
Incorporating Qualitative and Quantitative Evaluation Methods ........... 262
Gathering Feedback and Adapting Best Practices ........... 263
Systematic Analysis of Feedback ........... 264
Adapting Best Practices ........... 264
Continuous Education and Training for Ethics Consultants ........... 265
Fostering a Culture of Lifelong Learning ........... 265
Evaluating Training Effectiveness ........... 266
Ensuring Compliance and Upholding Ethical Standards ........... 266
12.1 Consultation Process Evaluation Template ........... 268
12.2 Stakeholder Feedback Collection Form ........... 270
12.3 Continuous Education and Training Plan ........... 272
Further Readings and References ........... 274

**Chapter 13: Personal and Professional Growth ........... 277**
Staying Informed on Regulatory Standards and Ethical Norms ........... 277
Promoting a Culture of Continuous Learning and Improvement: ........... 278
Tracking and Disseminating Updates ........... 278
Participating in Professional Conferences and Continuing Education ........... 279
Developing a Strategic Plan for Conference Engagement ........... 279
Encouraging Team Participation ........... 280
Implementing Organizational Policies for Work-life Balance ........... 281
Leading by Example ........... 282
13.1 Regulatory Standards and Ethical Norms Tracking Template ........... 284
13.2 Professional Development and Continuing Education Plan ........... 286
13.3 Work-Life Balance Assessment Template ........... 288
Further Readings and References ........... 290

**Chapter 14: Leading with Integrity and Compassion ........... 293**
Ethical Leadership in Healthcare ........... 293
Promoting Ethical Leadership Within the Organization ........... 294
Ongoing Self-reflection and Personal Growth ........... 294
Advocating for Ethical Practices ........... 295
Building Trust and Credibility ........... 295
Promoting a Culture of Trust and Credibility ........... 296
Transparency in Decision-Making ........... 296
Leading by Example and Inspiring Others ........... 296
Inspiring a Shared Vision ........... 297
Recognizing and Celebrating Contributions ........... 297

14.1 Stakeholder Trust-Building Checklist ....299
14.2 Recognition and Inspiration Log ....302
Further Readings and References ....304

**Review Questions ....307**

**Part VI: Practical Tools and Resources ....311**

**Chapter 15: Practical Tools for Bioethics Program Directors ....311**
Templates and Checklists for Policy Development ....311
Enhancing Quality and Consistency ....312
SOAP Notes and Documentation Guidelines ....313
Importance of Comprehensive Documentation ....314
Training and Support for Effective Documentation ....314
Promoting the Use of SOAP Notes ....315
Resources for Ethics Education and Training ....315
Interactive and Engaging Training Methods ....316
Promoting the Use of Educational Resources ....316
15.1/5.1 Policy Development Template ....318
15.2/5.2 Policy Development, Review, and Revision Checklist ....321
15.3 SOAP Notes ....324
— (S) Subjective ....324
— (O) Objective ....325
— (A) Assessment ....326
— (P) Plan ....326
15.4 Documentation Guidelines ....328
Further Readings and References ....329

**Chapter 16: Case Studies and Clinical Vignettes ....331**
The Value of Real-world Examples of Complex Ethical Dilemmas ....331
Incorporating Case Studies into Training ....332
Promoting the Use of Case Studies ....333
Interprofessional Approach to Ethics Education ....333
Facilitating Discussions and Reflections ....334
Lessons Learned and Best Practices ....335
Staying Informed About Emerging Trends ....336
Promoting a Culture of Continuous Learning ....336
16.1 Case Study Template ....338
16.2 Clinical Vignette Template ....340
16.3 Lessons Learned and Best Practices Summary ....342
Further Readings and References ....343

**Chapter 17: The Future of Bioethics Program Leadership ....345**
Staying Informed About Emerging Ethical Issues ....345
Navigating Emerging Technologies ....346
Adapting to Changes in Healthcare Regulations ....346
Addressing Evolving Societal Values ....347
Expanding the Scope and Reach of the Bioethics Program ....348
Promoting a Culture of Ethical Awareness and Responsibility ....348
Leading the Evolution of Bioethics in Healthcare ....349
Modeling Ethical Behavior ....350

Communicating Openly and Honestly....350
Treating All Stakeholders with Respect and Dignity....350
Inspiring Others....350
A Vision for the Future....351
17.1 Emerging Technologies Ethical Impact Assessment Template....352
17.2 Regulatory Changes Adaptation Plan Template....354
17.3 Stakeholder Engagement Plan Template....356
Further Readings and References....358

**Review Questions....361**

**Appendix:....365**

**Templates, Checklists, and Assessments....365**

**Glossary....375**

**Author....425**

**Notes....427**

# Volume 2: THE BIOETHICS Program Director's HANDBOOK
## Leading with Integrity and Compassion

---

# Part I: Understanding the Role of a Bioethics Program Director

---

## Chapter 1: Introduction to Bioethics Program Leadership

---

### Defining Bioethics

Bioethics is an interdisciplinary field that addresses ethical issues arising in healthcare, medicine, and the life sciences. It encompasses a wide range of topics, including patient rights, informed consent, end-of-life care, and the ethical implications of medical research and technologies. The core mission of bioethics is to ensure that patient care is both ethically justified and medically sound, which requires a nuanced understanding of the four foundational principles of bioethics: patient autonomy (informed consent), practitioner beneficence (maximize benefits), practitioner nonmaleficence (minimize burdens), and public justice (ensure fairness).

These principles are not static; they must be interpreted and applied in various contexts, such as clinical practice, research, and policy development. As a Bioethics Program Director, it is crucial to ensure that ethical decision-making is always guided by these principles while also adhering to professional medical standards of care, institutional policies, and legal mandates. The ultimate goal is to maximize the patient's best interests by aligning treatment options with the patient's reasonable goals, values, and priorities.

## Bioethical Principles

In the realm of bioethics, no single principle dominates; rather, each principle—patient autonomy (informed consent), practitioner beneficence (maximize benefits), practitioner nonmaleficence (minimize burdens), and public justice (ensure fairness)—must be specified, weighed, and balanced according to the circumstances at hand. This approach respects the patient's reasonable goals, values, and priorities while ensuring compliance with medical healthcare standards of care, institutional policies, and legal mandates.

**Patient Autonomy** (Informed Consent)

While patient autonomy is a fundamental component of ethical healthcare, it must be understood within the boundaries set by medical standards of care, institutional policies, and legal frameworks. Patient autonomy emphasizes the right of patients to be involved in their healthcare decisions. However, this right is not absolute and should be exercised within the options provided by healthcare practitioners, which align with established medical standards of care, and do not violate institutional policies or legal mandates. The role of the Bioethics Program Director is to ensure that the principle of autonomy is respected by facilitating informed consent.

Informed consent requires that patients, or their legally established surrogates when patients lack decisional capacity, fully understand their diagnosis and prognosis, are aware of all medically appropriate treatment options (including the option of no treatment), comprehend the purpose of each proposed intervention, and can evaluate the potential benefits and risks involved. Patients and surrogates must be able to articulate logical reasons for their healthcare choices, reflecting their reasonable goals, values, and priorities. This decision-making process should always be guided by the ethicist's role in specifying, weighing, and balancing the principle of autonomy alongside the principles of nonmaleficence (minimize burdens), beneficence (maximize benefits), and public justice (ensure fairness). By doing so, ethical decisions are made that align with the patient's best interests within the scope of professional practice.

**Practitioner Beneficence** (Maximize Benefits)

Beneficence involves actively contributing to the well-being of the patient. The Bioethics Program Director must advocate for treatments that not only meet clinical effectiveness but also align with the patient's reasonable goals, values, and priorities. Practitioners are ethically obligated to propose options that maximize benefits, minimize potential harms, and improve the patient's overall quality of life. This requires a holistic view of care that goes beyond immediate medical outcomes, encompassing the patient's broader psychosocial well-being.

The principle of beneficence must be balanced with the principles of patient autonomy, nonmaleficence, and public justice. The Bioethics Program Director's role is to guide practitioners in considering how proposed treatments align with the patient's preferences and how these treatments adhere to medical healthcare standards of care, and ethical principles. This ensures that beneficence is pursued not in isolation but as part of a comprehensive ethical approach that respects the patient's values and legal rights.

**Practitioner Nonmaleficence** (Minimize Burdens)

The principle of nonmaleficence, the obligation to avoid causing harm, is a cornerstone of ethical medical practice. Nonmaleficence requires healthcare providers to take proactive steps to minimize risks and prevent harm to patients. This principle demands thorough risk assessments and the consideration of potential negative outcomes associated with any treatment or intervention.

Nonmaleficence does not operate in a vacuum; it must be balanced with the principles of patient autonomy, beneficence, and justice. For example, a patient's autonomous decision to refuse a life-saving treatment must be respected if it aligns with their informed understanding and personal goals, values, and priorities. The Bioethics Program Director's role is to ensure that decisions are made with a focus on minimizing harm while considering the patient's rights, the promotion of benefits, and the fair distribution of healthcare resources.

**Public Justice** (Ensure Fairness)

Public justice emphasizes the fair and equitable treatment of all patients and the ethical distribution of healthcare resources. It involves ensuring that healthcare decisions do not disadvantage vulnerable populations and that access to care is fair and just. The Bioethics Program Director must advocate for policies and practices that address healthcare disparities, promote equitable access to care, and protect the rights of marginalized groups.

Justice in bioethics requires balancing the needs of the individual patient with the broader needs of society. Decisions should be made with an awareness of their impact on both the immediate patient and the larger community, ensuring that ethical principles are applied consistently and fairly. The Bioethics Program Director's role includes facilitating a healthcare environment where justice informs both clinical and administrative decisions, contributing to an overall ethical culture that values fairness and equity.

## The Role of the Bioethics Program Director

The Bioethics Program Director serves as a pivotal figure in ensuring that all four core bioethical principles are integrated into healthcare decision-making. By guiding the specifying, weighing, and balancing of patient autonomy (informed consent), practitioner beneficence (maximize benefits), practitioner nonmaleficence (minimize burdens), and public justice (ensure fairness), the director ensures that patient care aligns with ethical standards, medical standards, and legal standards. This role involves continuous dialogue with healthcare providers, patients, and other stakeholders to navigate complex ethical dilemmas and uphold the mission and vision of the Bioethics Program. The director's leadership in these areas fosters a healthcare environment where ethical considerations are central to every decision, promoting integrity, compassion, and justice in patient care.

### Compliance and Continuous Ethical Education

Ensuring compliance with the principles of bioethics, as well as with established medical standards, institutional policies, and legal mandates, is critical to the role of the Bioethics Program Director. This includes promoting ethical awareness, understanding, and continuous education among healthcare practitioners and ethics consultants. Continuous education is vital for keeping abreast of evolving ethical debates, legal standards, and emerging issues in bioethics. The director should facilitate ongoing training, participation in bioethics conferences, and engagement with the broader bioethics community to ensure that ethical considerations are integrated into every aspect of patient care and decision-making.

### Role and Responsibilities of a Bioethics Program Director

The Bioethics Program Director plays a central role in maintaining and advancing ethical standards within a healthcare organization. Key responsibilities include providing leadership and oversight for the Bioethics Program, conducting healthcare ethics consultations, and developing and implementing ethical policies. The director must also engage in preventive ethics activities, which involve identifying and addressing potential ethical issues before they escalate. This can be achieved through routine ethics audits, creating early warning systems for ethical breaches, and fostering an environment where practitioners feel comfortable raising ethical concerns.

Effective leadership requires a deep understanding of both clinical practices and ethical principles. The Bioethics Program Director must be skilled in communication and mediation, able to navigate complex ethical dilemmas, and provide clear, well-reasoned guidance. Crisis management skills are essential, as ethical dilemmas often arise unexpectedly and require immediate attention. Ensuring that the outcomes of ethics consultations are documented and reviewed is crucial for accountability, training, and continuous improvement of ethical practices.

## Integrating Ethical Principles in Leadership

The director's role extends to advocating for the integration of ethical principles into all aspects of the healthcare organization. This involves working with senior leadership to embed these principles into the organization's mission, vision, and strategic goals. By aligning the Bioethics Program with the broader organizational objectives, the director can promote a culture of ethical awareness and accountability, ensuring that ethical considerations are integrated into every decision made by patients, surrogates, and practitioners.

Interdisciplinary collaboration is crucial for addressing complex ethical issues that span multiple areas of expertise. The Bioethics Program Director must work with physicians, nurses, social workers, legal experts, and other healthcare professionals to ensure that ethical decisions are well-informed and consider all relevant perspectives and factors. This collaborative approach enhances the quality of ethical deliberations and promotes a holistic understanding of the ethical issues at hand.

## Key Skills and Qualities for Effective Leadership

An effective Bioethics Program Director must possess a unique blend of skills and qualities. Strong interpersonal and communication skills are essential for facilitating discussions, mediating conflicts, and educating practitioners. Analytical and critical thinking skills are vital for assessing complex ethical dilemmas and developing sound recommendations. Organizational skills are necessary for managing multiple projects, coordinating activities, and ensuring compliance with ethical and regulatory standards.

Leadership and decision-making abilities are crucial, particularly in high-pressure situations. The director must be able to prioritize issues, delegate tasks, and make difficult decisions when necessary. Mentorship and the development of other bioethics team members are also key responsibilities, ensuring that they are equipped to handle ethical issues independently. This mentorship can take the form of regular training sessions, one-on-one coaching, and providing opportunities for professional development.

A commitment to ethical principles and integrity is vital, as is adaptability and a dedication to life-long learning. The dynamic nature of bioethics requires staying current with the latest developments, which can be achieved through continuous professional development, participation in bioethics conferences, and engagement with academic and professional networks. Problem-solving skills and the ability to think creatively are also essential, enabling the director to address the diverse and evolving ethical challenges in healthcare.

## Conclusion

The Bioethics Program Director plays a central role in upholding and advancing the ethical standards within a healthcare organization. By aligning the Bioethics Program with the organization's mission and vision, the director ensures that ethical considerations are integrated into patient care, policy development, and education. Through the application of the core bioethical principles—patient autonomy (informed consent), practitioner beneficence (maximize benefits), practitioner nonmaleficence (minimize burdens), and public justice (ensure fairness)—the director promotes an ethical culture that prioritizes the patient's best interests, supports fair and equitable treatment, and adheres to the highest standards of care, institutional policies, and legal requirements. By fostering a commitment to ethical reflection, dialogue, and continuous education, the Bioethics Program Director ensures that both patients and surrogates are fully informed, enabling well-reasoned decisions that enhance the quality and compassion of patient care.

***

The following forms and templates are essential tools for Bioethics Program Directors, providing a structured approach to organizing their responsibilities, tracking progress, and ensuring that their roles are executed effectively. By utilizing these resources, directors can maintain clarity and consistency in their work, identify areas for improvement, and support their ongoing development.

***

## 1.1 Leadership Self-Assessment Tool

---

**Purpose:** To help the Bioethics Program Director regularly assess their ethical leadership practices, competencies, and identify areas for personal and professional growth.

**Name:** [Name of Director]
**Date:** [Date of Self-Assessment]
**Department:** [Department Name]

**Instructions:**
Rate your proficiency in each area using the scale provided, and reflect on your strengths. Use the provided space to offer examples where applicable and identify areas where further development is needed.

---

**Competency Area 1: Integrity and Ethical Decision-Making**

- **Integrity in Decision-Making:**
  Do I consistently demonstrate integrity in all my decisions and actions?
  Rating (1-5): [ ]
  [Comments/Examples]
- **Ethical Decision-Making:**
  Do I make ethical decisions based on a thorough understanding of ethical principles and organizational values?
  Rating (1-5): [ ]
  [Comments/Examples]
- **Transparency in Decision-Making:**
  Am I transparent in my decision-making process, and do I communicate the rationale behind my decisions to stakeholders?
  Rating (1-5): [ ]
  [Comments/Examples]

---

**Competency Area 2: Understanding of Bioethical Principles**

- **Patient Autonomy** (Informed Consent):
  Rating (1-5): [ ]
  [Examples of how you have applied this principle in your work]
- **Practitioner Beneficence** (Maximize Benefits):
  Rating (1-5): [ ]
  [Examples of how you have applied this principle in your work]
- **Practitioner Nonmaleficence** (Minimize Burdens):
  Rating (1-5): [ ]
  [Examples of how you have applied this principle in your work]
- **Public Justice** (Ensure Fairness):
  Rating (1-5): [ ]
  [Examples of how you have applied this principle in your work]

---

**Competency Area 3: Leadership and Decision-Making**

- **Crisis Management:**
  Rating (1-5): [ ]
  [Describe a situation where you successfully managed a crisis]
- **Delegation:**
  Rating (1-5): [ ]
  [Describe how you delegate tasks within your team]
- **Mentorship:**
  Rating (1-5): [ ]
  [Examples of how you have mentored team members]

---

**Competency Area 4: Transparency and Accountability**

- **Personal Accountability:**
  Do I hold myself accountable for my actions and decisions?

Rating (1-5): [ ]
[Comments/Examples]

- **Encouraging Team Accountability:**
  Do I encourage accountability among my team members?
  Rating (1-5): [ ]
  [Comments/Examples]
- **Open Communication:**
  Am I open and honest in my communication with others?
  Rating (1-5): [ ]
  [Comments/Examples]

---

**Competency Area 5: Interpersonal and Communication Skills**

- **Empathy and Compassion:**
  Do I demonstrate empathy and compassion in my interactions with others?
  Rating (1-5): [ ]
  [Comments/Examples]
- **Active Listening:**
  Do I actively listen to the concerns and perspectives of others?
  Rating (1-5): [ ]
  [Comments/Examples]
- **Facilitating Ethical Discussions:**
  Rating (1-5): [ ]
  [Provide an example of a successful ethical discussion you facilitated]
- **Conflict Mediation:**
  Rating (1-5): [ ]
  [Describe a time you effectively mediated a conflict]

---

**Competency Area 6: Analytical and Critical Thinking**

- **Assessing Complex Ethical Dilemmas:**
  Rating (1-5): [ ]
  [Provide an example of a complex ethical dilemma you assessed and the outcome]

- **Ethical Decision-Making Process:**
  Rating (1-5): [ ]
  [Describe how you incorporate ethical principles into your decision-making process]
- **Innovation and Problem Solving:**
  Rating (1-5): [ ]
  [Give an example of a creative solution you developed for an ethical issue]

---

**Competency Area 7: Organizational and Administrative Skills**

- **Project Management:**
  Rating (1-5): [ ]
  [Describe your approach to managing multiple projects]
- **Policy Development:**
  Rating (1-5): [ ]
  [Provide an example of a policy you developed or revised]
- **Compliance with Regulatory Standards:**
  Rating (1-5): [ ]
  [Describe how you ensure compliance within your organization]

---

**Competency Area 8: Inspiring and Motivating Others**

- **Communicating Vision and Goals:**
  Do I effectively communicate the vision and goals of the Bioethics Program?
  Rating (1-5): [ ]
  [Comments/Examples]
- **Recognition and Celebration:**
  Do I recognize and celebrate the contributions of team members?
  Rating (1-5): [ ]
  [Comments/Examples]
- **Inspiring Ethical Practice:**
  Do I inspire others to uphold ethical principles and practices?

Rating (1-5): [ ]
[Comments/Examples]

---

**Competency Area 9: Personal Development and Lifelong Learning**

- **Commitment to Lifelong Learning:**
  Rating (1-5): [ ]
  [List recent professional development activities (e.g., conferences, courses)]
- **Adaptability to New Ethical Challenges:**
  Rating (1-5): [ ]
  [Describe how you stay current with emerging ethical issues in healthcare]

---

**Overall Reflection**

- **Strengths:**
  Identify your key strengths as a Bioethics Program Director.
  [Provide details]
- **Areas for Growth and Development:**
  What areas do you need to work on to improve your leadership?
  [List specific areas for improvement]
- **Action Plan:**
  *What steps will you take to improve in these areas?*
  [Outline a plan for personal and professional growth]

---

**Next Review Date:** [Date] Set a date for the next self-assessment.

***

## 1.2 Ethical Dilemma Case Documentation Form

**Purpose**: To document ethical dilemmas encountered in the healthcare setting, ensuring that they are analyzed, resolved, and reviewed systematically.

**Case ID**: [Unique Case Identifier]
**Date of Consultation**: [Date]
**Consultant(s)**: [Name(s) of Ethics Consultant(s)]

**Case Overview**:

- Provide a brief summary of the case, including relevant clinical and ethical details. [Enter details]

**Ethical Issues**:

- Identify the primary ethical issues involved in the case (e.g., patient autonomy, confidentiality, informed consent). [Enter details]

**Stakeholder Perspectives**:

- Summarize the perspectives of the key stakeholders (e.g., patient, family, healthcare team). [Enter details]

**Ethical Principles Applied**:

- Describe the ethical principles that are relevant to the case and how they apply. [Enter details]

**Analysis and Discussion**:

- Detail the ethical analysis conducted, including consideration of various perspectives, principles, and possible courses of action. [Enter details]

**Recommended Course of Action**:

- Provide the recommended resolution or course of action, including the rationale behind the decision. [Enter details]

**Outcome**:

- Document the outcome of the case, including how the recommended actions were implemented and the final resolution. [Enter details]

**Follow-Up**:

- List any follow-up actions required (e.g., further consultations, policy revisions) and assign responsibility. [Enter details]

**Reflection**:

- Reflect on the case and its implications for future practice. What were the key takeaways, and how can they inform future decisions? [Enter details]

**Signatures**:

- Consultant(s) Signature: [Signature]
- Date: [Date]

***

## 1.3 Ethics Program Development Checklist

**Purpose**: To guide the Bioethics Program Director through the essential steps of developing or refining a Bioethics Program, ensuring that all critical elements are addressed.

**Date of Review**: [Date]
**Reviewed by**: [Name of Director or Team Member]

**Program Foundations**

- ☐ Mission Statement: Clearly defined and aligned with organizational values.
- ☐ Vision Statement: Articulates long-term goals and ethical aspirations.
- ☐ Values Statement: Outlines core ethical principles guiding the program.

**Program Structure**

- ☐ Ethics Committee: Established with diverse representation from relevant disciplines.
- ☐ Consultation Services: Procedures for providing timely and effective ethics consultations.
- ☐ Policy Development: Framework for creating and reviewing ethical policies.
- ☐ Education and Training: Regular ethics education programs for staff and stakeholders.
- ☐ Preventive Ethics Activities: Initiatives for identifying and addressing ethical issues proactively.

**Operational Elements**

- ☐ Documentation and Record-Keeping: System for documenting consultations and decisions.
- ☐ Compliance with Legal Standards: Regular review to ensure alignment with relevant laws and regulations.
- ☐ Interdisciplinary Collaboration: Mechanisms for working with other departments and experts.
- ☐ Evaluation and Improvement: Regular assessment of program effectiveness and areas for enhancement.

**Community and Professional Engagement**

- ☐ Outreach Activities: Engagement with the broader community and professional organizations.
- ☐ Public Education: Initiatives for raising public awareness about bioethics.
- ☐ Research and Scholarship: Opportunities for contributing to the field through research and publications.

**Program Review and Future Planning**

- ☐ Regular Program Review: Scheduled evaluations of the program's effectiveness and relevance.
- ☐ Strategic Planning: Long-term goals and strategies for program growth and impact.
- ☐ Resource Allocation: Ensuring adequate resources (staff, budget, etc.) to sustain program activities.

**Final Review**

- ☐ All elements addressed and verified: [ ]
- ☐ Next review date scheduled: [ ]
- ☐ Signatures of reviewers and date: [ ]

***

## 1.4 Stakeholder Engagement Template

**Purpose**: To plan and track engagement with key stakeholders, ensuring that their perspectives are considered in bioethics program decisions and initiatives.

**Date of Engagement**: [Date]
**Stakeholder Name/Group**: [Name of Stakeholder or Group]

**Role/Interest in Bioethics Program**

- Describe the stakeholder's role or interest in the program (e.g., patient advocate, clinical department head, legal advisor). [Enter details]

**Objectives for Engagement**

- Outline the objectives for engaging with this stakeholder (e.g., gather input on policy development, collaborate on ethics education). [Enter details]

**Engagement Activities**

- List the planned activities for engagement (e.g., meetings, surveys, focus groups). [Enter details]

**Key Discussion Points**

- Summarize the key points discussed during the engagement activities. [Enter details]

**Stakeholder Feedback**

- Document any feedback, concerns, or suggestions provided by the stakeholder. [Enter details]

**Action Items**

- List any follow-up actions or decisions resulting from the engagement, including responsibilities and deadlines. [Enter details]

**Outcome**

- Describe the outcome of the engagement and how it will inform the bioethics program's activities. [Enter details]

**Next Steps**

- Outline the next steps for maintaining or furthering engagement with this stakeholder. [Enter details]

**Signatures**

- Engagement Lead: [Signature]
- Date: [Date]

***

## 1.5 Program Director's Monthly Report Template

**Purpose**: To document and report on the monthly activities, challenges, and achievements of the Bioethics Program, ensuring accountability and transparency.

**Month/Year**: [Month/Year]
**Prepared by**: [Name of Director]

**I. Overview of Activities**

- Provide a summary of key activities and initiatives undertaken during the month (e.g., ethics consultations, policy development, education programs). [Enter details]

**II. Key Accomplishments**

- Highlight major achievements or milestones reached (e.g., successful resolution of a complex case, completion of a new policy). [Enter details]

**III. Challenges Encountered**

- Describe any significant challenges faced and how they were addressed (e.g., ethical conflicts, resource constraints). [Enter details]

**IV. Stakeholder Engagement**

- Provide an overview of stakeholder engagement activities (e.g., meetings, collaborations, outreach efforts). [Enter details]

**V. Preventive Ethics Initiatives**

- Summarize preventive ethics activities, including any early warning systems activated or issues preemptively addressed. [Enter details]

**VI. Education and Training**

- Provide a summary of ethics education programs delivered and participant feedback. [Enter details]

**VII. Program Development and Evaluation**

- Report on progress with program development initiatives, including any evaluations or improvements made. [Enter details]

**VIII. Upcoming Activities**

- Outline planned activities for the upcoming month, including any important dates or deadlines. [Enter details]

**IX. Resource Needs**

- Identify any resource needs or requests (e.g., additional staff, budget adjustments, training materials). [Enter details]

**X. Additional Comments**

- Include any other relevant information or reflections. [Enter details]

**Signatures**

- Director's Signature: [Signature]
- Date: [Date]

***

# Further Readings and References


## Defining Bioethics

- Beauchamp, T. L., & Childress, J. F. (2013). Principles of Biomedical Ethics (7th ed.). Oxford University Press.
  - *A foundational text that outlines the core principles of biomedical ethics: autonomy, beneficence, nonmaleficence, and justice. It provides a comprehensive framework for ethical decision-making in healthcare.*
- Gillon, R. (1994). Medical ethics: four principles plus attention to scope. BMJ, 309(6948), 184-188.
  - *An influential article that emphasizes the application of the four principles approach in medical ethics and discusses the importance of considering the scope of ethical issues.*
- Jonsen, A. R., Siegler, M., & Winslade, W. J. (2010). Clinical Ethics: A Practical Approach to Ethical Decisions in Clinical Medicine (7th ed.). McGraw-Hill Education.
  - *This practical guide addresses real-world clinical ethical dilemmas and provides a structured approach to ethical decision-making in clinical settings.*

## The Role and Responsibilities of a Bioethics Program Director

- Glasa, J. (Ed.). (2015). Medical Ethics Education: An Interdisciplinary and Social Theoretical Perspective. Springer.
  - *Explores the interdisciplinary nature of medical ethics education and its implications for the role of a bioethics program director in fostering ethical awareness and decision-making.*
- Heubel, F. (2005). The role of clinical ethics committees in clinical decision-making. Medicine, Health Care and Philosophy, 8(2), 155-157.
  - *Discusses the critical function of clinical ethics committees in guiding ethical decisions in healthcare institutions and the*

*leadership role of bioethics program directors in these committees.*

- Shapiro, J. P. (2011). Ethical Leadership and Decision Making in Education: Applying Theoretical Perspectives to Complex Dilemmas (3rd ed.). Routledge.
  - *Analyzes ethical leadership theories and their application to educational settings, providing insights into the leadership skills necessary for a bioethics program director.*

**Key Skills and Qualities for Effective Leadership**

- Gini, A., & Green, R. M. (2013). Ten Virtues of Outstanding Leaders: Leadership and Character. Wiley-Blackwell.
  - *Identifies and discusses the essential virtues and character traits that define exceptional leaders, relevant for those leading bioethics programs.*
- Northouse, P. G. (2018). Leadership: Theory and Practice (8th ed.). Sage Publications.
  - *A comprehensive examination of various leadership theories and practices, offering valuable perspectives for bioethics program directors to enhance their leadership effectiveness.*
- Yukl, G. A. (2012). Leadership in Organizations (8th ed.). Pearson.
  - *Explores leadership strategies and their impact on organizational effectiveness, providing practical guidance for bioethics program directors.*

***

# Chapter 2: Building a Strong Foundation

A successful Bioethics Program must align its initiatives with the strategic goals of the healthcare organization. This alignment is essential to ensure that ethical considerations are integrated into every aspect of healthcare delivery, enhancing patient care and organizational integrity. It involves understanding the institution's mission, vision, and values, and ensuring that bioethics activities support these objectives.

## Integrating Bioethics with Organizational Strategy

To achieve strategic alignment, the Bioethics Program Director must actively participate in strategic planning meetings and collaborate closely with senior leadership. This collaboration is critical to ensure that ethical perspectives are considered in all major decisions. It involves:

1. **Participating in Strategic Planning:** The director should be involved in strategic planning to advocate for the integration of ethical considerations into organizational goals. This includes participating in discussions on clinical priorities, resource allocation, and policy development to ensure that ethical values are upheld.
2. **Developing Strategic Partnerships:** Building partnerships with key stakeholders, such as department heads, senior executives, and legal advisors, is vital. These partnerships help create alignment between clinical and ethical priorities, ensuring that the organization's strategic goals reflect its commitment to ethical practice.
3. **Advocating for Ethical Resource Allocation:** Ethical considerations should influence how resources are allocated within the organization. This includes advocating for budget allocations that support ethical initiatives, such as ethics

consultation services, staff training, and research into emerging ethical issues.

4. **Embedding Ethical Considerations in Decision-Making:** By embedding ethical considerations into decision-making processes, the Bioethics Program can help ensure that ethical principles guide all organizational activities. This can involve creating ethical checklists for decision-making, ensuring that ethical impact assessments are conducted for new initiatives, and establishing protocols for addressing ethical dilemmas.

## Evaluating and Communicating the Impact of Bioethics Initiatives

The Bioethics Program Director should establish metrics and evaluation processes to assess the impact of bioethics initiatives on organizational goals. Regular assessments help identify areas for improvement, demonstrate the value of the Bioethics Program, and provide data to support ongoing investment in ethical initiatives. The evaluation process should include:

1. **Defining Key Performance Indicators (KPIs):** KPIs for bioethics initiatives might include the number of ethics consultations conducted, practitioner satisfaction with ethics support, patient outcomes related to ethical decision-making, and compliance with ethical guidelines.
2. **Conducting Regular Evaluations:** Regular evaluations of the Bioethics Program's activities help ensure that they are effective and aligned with organizational goals. This can involve surveys, feedback sessions, and audits to gather data on the program's impact.
3. **Communicating Value to Stakeholders:** The director must effectively communicate the value of the Bioethics Program to senior leadership and other stakeholders. This can be achieved through regular reports, presentations, and meetings, highlighting how bioethics activities contribute to improving

patient care, enhancing practitioner satisfaction, and reducing legal risks.

## Integrating Bioethics into All Organizational Levels

To ensure that ethical considerations are consistently applied across the organization, bioethics initiatives must be integrated at all levels. This involves:

1. **Collaborating with Department Heads:** The director should work with department heads to identify and address ethical issues specific to their areas of practice. This collaboration helps tailor bioethics initiatives to meet the unique needs of different departments.
2. **Empowering Frontline Practitioners:** Frontline practitioners play a crucial role in upholding ethical standards. The director should provide resources, training, and support to help them recognize and navigate ethical dilemmas. This can include access to ethical guidelines, decision-making frameworks, and consultation services.
3. **Fostering a Culture of Ethical Awareness:** By promoting a culture of ethical awareness and responsibility, the director can help ensure that ethical principles are consistently applied in patient care and decision-making. This involves creating an environment where ethical concerns can be openly discussed and addressed.

## Establishing and Leading the Bioethics Committee

The Bioethics Committee is a vital component of the Bioethics Program, providing a forum for addressing ethical issues and supporting ethical decision-making in clinical practice. The director's role includes:

1. **Recruiting and Training Committee Members:** A strong Bioethics Committee should be diverse and interprofessional, reflecting the perspectives of various stakeholders, including physicians, nurses, social workers, and patient representatives.

The director must ensure that committee members are well-trained and equipped to address complex ethical issues.

2. **Facilitating Effective Meetings:** The director should facilitate regular committee meetings, creating a structured environment where ethical issues can be discussed openly. This involves preparing agendas, guiding discussions, and ensuring that decisions are well-documented and communicated to relevant stakeholders.
3. **Providing Ongoing Education:** Ongoing education is essential to keep committee members informed about current ethical issues and best practices. The director should organize training sessions, workshops, and seminars to enhance the committee's effectiveness.
4. **Ensuring Access to Resources:** The committee must have access to the necessary resources and support to perform its duties effectively. This includes access to ethical guidelines, legal expertise, and educational materials. By empowering the committee with the tools they need, the director can enhance their ability to address ethical issues proactively.
5. **Promoting Informal Interactions:** In addition to formal meetings, the director should encourage informal interactions among committee members. These interactions can help build trust and foster a collaborative environment, enhancing the committee's effectiveness.

## Creating a Culture of Ethical Sensitivity and Collaboration

Fostering a culture of ethical sensitivity and collaboration is essential for integrating ethical considerations into everyday clinical practice. The director should promote:

1. **Open Communication:** Encourage open communication where practitioners feel comfortable raising ethical concerns. This involves creating safe spaces for dialogue, such as ethics cafés

or discussion groups, where practitioners can share experiences and perspectives.

2. **Ethical Reflection:** Support ethical reflection by providing opportunities for practitioners to reflect on their experiences and consider the ethical dimensions of their practice. This can include ethics rounds, case discussions, and reflective practice sessions.
3. **Interdisciplinary Collaboration:** Promote interdisciplinary collaboration to address complex ethical issues. This can involve regular interdisciplinary meetings, joint training sessions, and collaborative projects that bring together practitioners from different disciplines to discuss and address ethical issues.
4. **Recognizing and Rewarding Ethical Behavior:** Establish mechanisms for recognizing and rewarding ethical behavior. This can involve creating awards or incentives for practitioners who demonstrate exceptional ethical judgment and integrity. By celebrating ethical behavior, the director can reinforce the importance of ethics and encourage others to follow suit.
5. **Continuous Education and Development:** Implement regular training sessions, workshops, and seminars to keep practitioners informed about ethical issues. These educational activities should be interactive and relevant, allowing practitioners to discuss real-world cases and explore ethical dilemmas in a supportive environment.

## Implementing Ethical Guidelines and Protocols

The Bioethics Program Director should ensure that clear ethical guidelines and protocols are established and implemented across the organization. These guidelines should:

1. **Provide Clear Guidance:** Offer clear guidance on how to handle common ethical issues, such as informed consent, confidentiality, end-of-life care, and resource allocation. These guidelines should be accessible to all practitioners and regularly updated to reflect current best practices.

2. **Support Decision-Making:** Ethical protocols should support practitioners in making ethical decisions. This can involve creating ethical decision-making frameworks, providing consultation services, and offering tools for ethical analysis.
3. **Ensure Compliance with Standards:** Ethical guidelines must align with established medical standards of care, institutional policies, and legal mandates. The director should work with legal and compliance teams to ensure that ethical protocols are compliant with all relevant regulations.
4. **Promote Consistency:** Consistency is key to maintaining ethical standards. The director should ensure that ethical guidelines are consistently applied across the organization, providing training and support to help practitioners understand and implement these guidelines.

**Conclusion**

Building a strong foundation for a Bioethics Program involves aligning bioethics initiatives with the strategic goals of the healthcare organization, establishing and leading an effective Bioethics Committee, and fostering a culture of ethical sensitivity and collaboration. By integrating the core bioethical principles—patient autonomy (informed consent), practitioner beneficence (maximize benefits), practitioner nonmaleficence (minimize burdens), and public justice (ensure fairness)—into all aspects of healthcare delivery, the Bioethics Program Director can enhance the ethical quality of patient care and support the organization's mission and vision. Through strategic planning, collaboration, education, and the implementation of clear ethical guidelines, the director ensures that ethical considerations are embedded in the fabric of the healthcare system, promoting a commitment to integrity, compassion, and excellence in patient care.

***

The following forms and templates are designed to provide a comprehensive framework for building a strong foundation for Bioethics Programs, ensuring alignment with organizational goals, effective committee operations, and fostering a culture of ethical sensitivity and collaboration.

***

## 2.1 Strategic Alignment Checklist

**Purpose**: To ensure that the Bioethics Program aligns with the organization's strategic goals and objectives.

**Date**: [Date]
**Completed by**: [Name]

**Mission and Vision Alignment**

- ☐ Reviewed the organization's mission, vision, and values.
- ☐ Ensured the Bioethics Program's mission and vision support organizational goals.
- ☐ Identified specific ways bioethics initiatives contribute to the organization's objectives.

**Strategic Planning Participation**

- ☐ Participated in strategic planning meetings with senior leadership.
- ☐ Advocated for ethical considerations in organizational decision-making processes.
- ☐ Established partnerships with key stakeholders to integrate ethics into strategic initiatives.

**Ethical Impact Metrics**

- ☐ Developed metrics to evaluate the impact of bioethics initiatives on organizational goals.
- ☐ Conducted regular assessments of bioethics activities to ensure alignment with strategic goals.
- ☐ Used data from evaluations to adjust and improve bioethics initiatives.

**Communication with Leadership**

- ☐ Prepared regular reports for senior leadership highlighting the value of bioethics activities.
- ☐ Presented bioethics contributions to organizational goals in meetings or presentations.
- ☐ Ensured ongoing dialogue with key stakeholders about the role of bioethics in achieving organizational objectives.

**Integration Across Organization**

- ☐ Collaborated with department heads to integrate ethical considerations into departmental strategies.
- ☐ Supported frontline practitioners in addressing ethical issues specific to their practice areas.
- ☐ Promoted ethical awareness and responsibility across all levels of the organization.

**Review and Continuous Improvement**

- ☐ Scheduled regular reviews of bioethics initiatives to ensure continued alignment with strategic goals.
- ☐ Updated bioethics strategies based on feedback from assessments and organizational changes.
- ☐ Engaged with stakeholders during reviews to maintain alignment and support for bioethics activities.

***

## 2.2 Bioethics Committee Member Selection Form

**Purpose**: To ensure a diverse, interprofessional Bioethics Committee that represents various perspectives and expertise.

**Date**: [Date]
**Completed by**: [Name of Director]
**Candidate Name**: [Name]
**Professional Background**: [Enter details about the candidate's profession (e.g., physician, nurse, social worker)]

**Qualifications**

- Relevant experience in bioethics: [Enter details]
- Previous committee work or leadership roles: [Enter details]
- Interdisciplinary collaboration experience: [Enter details]

**Representation**

- ☐ Reflects diverse perspectives relevant to bioethics (e.g., clinical, legal, patient advocacy).
- ☐ Contributes to the interprofessional nature of the committee.
- ☐ Brings unique insights or expertise to the committee's work.

**Availability and Commitment**

- ☐ Demonstrates willingness to commit to regular meetings and participation in committee activities.
- ☐ Available for ongoing education and development in bioethics.
- ☐ Willing to contribute to committee-led initiatives and projects.

**Potential Contribution**

- ☐ Expected to provide valuable input in bioethical discussions.
- ☐ Can help enhance the committee's effectiveness in addressing ethical issues.
- ☐ Likely to engage constructively with other committee members.

**Final Recommendation**

- ☐ Recommend for committee membership
- ☐ Do not recommend at this time

**Comments**: [Enter any additional comments]

**Signature of Director**: [Signature]
**Date**: [Date]

***

## 2.3 Bioethics Committee Meeting Agenda Template

**Purpose**: To organize and guide Bioethics Committee meetings, ensuring that all relevant issues are addressed efficiently.

**Date**: [Date]
**Time**: [Time]
**Location**: [Location]
**Facilitator**: [Name of Director]

**Welcome and Introductions**

- Brief introductions (if needed)
- Overview of the meeting's purpose

**Review of Previous Meeting Minutes**

- Summary of the last meeting's key points
- Approval of minutes

**Current Ethical Issues for Discussion**

- Case 1: [Brief description of the case]
- Discussion points
- Proposed resolutions
- Case 2: [Brief description of the case]
- Discussion points
- Proposed resolutions

**Policy Development and Updates**

- Review of new or revised policies
- Discussion on implementation strategies

**Education and Training Initiatives**

- Upcoming training sessions
- Feedback from recent training events

**Preventive Ethics Activities**

- Overview of proactive measures
- Discussion on early warning systems and their effectiveness

**Open Forum**

- Opportunity for committee members to raise new issues or concerns
- Discussion on any additional topics

**Summary of Action Items**

- Review of agreed-upon actions
- Assignment of responsibilities and deadlines

**Next Meeting**

- Date and time of the next meeting
- Preliminary agenda items

**Adjournment**

- Closing remarks
- Meeting adjourned

***

## 2.4 Ethical Sensitivity and Collaboration Action Plan

**Purpose**: To create a structured plan for promoting ethical sensitivity and collaboration across the organization.

**Date**: [Date]
**Prepared by**: [Name of Director]
**Objective**: To foster a culture of ethical sensitivity and interdisciplinary collaboration within the organization.

**Training and Education**

- ☐ Develop and schedule regular ethics training sessions.
  - Topics: [List topics (e.g., informed consent, end-of-life care)]
  - Target Audience: [Specify audience (e.g., clinical practitioners, administrative personnel)]
  - Resources Required: [List resources (e.g., trainers, materials)]
- ☐ Implement ethics rounds and workshops.
  - Frequency: [Enter frequency]
  - Facilitators: [List names]

**Informal Ethical Discussions**

- ☐ Establish ethics cafés or discussion groups.
  - Locations: [Enter locations]
  - Schedule: [Enter schedule]
- ☐ Promote a culture of open dialogue about ethical issues.
  - Communication Channels: [List channels (e.g., internal forums, newsletters)]
  - Participation Encouragement: [Describe strategies]

**Recognition of Ethical Behavior**

- ☐ Create awards or incentives for demonstrating ethical behavior.
  - ▸ Criteria: [Describe criteria]
  - ▸ Nomination Process: [Describe process]
- ☐ Highlight examples of ethical decision-making in organizational communications.
  - ▸ Methods: [List methods (e.g., newsletters, meetings)]

**Interdisciplinary Collaboration**

- ☐ Organize regular interdisciplinary meetings on ethical issues.
  - ▸ Participants: [List departments or roles]
  - ▸ Frequency: [Enter frequency]
- ☐ Facilitate joint training sessions for different disciplines.
  - ▸ Topics: [List topics]
  - ▸ Trainers: [List trainers]

**Evaluation and Continuous Improvement**

- ☐ Establish metrics to assess the effectiveness of ethical sensitivity initiatives.
  - ▸ Metrics: [Describe metrics]
  - ▸ Review Schedule: [Enter schedule]
- ☐ Collect feedback from participants and stakeholders.
  - ▸ Feedback Methods: [List methods (e.g., surveys, interviews)]
- ☐ Regularly update the action plan based on feedback and new developments.
  - ▸ Update Schedule: [Enter schedule]

**Director's Signature**: [Signature]
**Date**: [Date]

***

# Further Readings and References

## Aligning Bioethics Initiatives with Strategic Organizational Goals


- Kalb, P. E. (2012). Aligning bioethics programs with strategic goals. Health Care Ethics USA, 20(1), 1-7.
  - *Discusses strategies for aligning bioethics programs with the overarching strategic goals of healthcare organizations, emphasizing the importance of integration and support.*
- Pellegrino, E. D., & Thomasma, D. C. (1993). The Virtues in Medical Practice. Oxford University Press.
  - *Examines the role of virtues in medical practice and their relevance to bioethics, providing a philosophical foundation for aligning bioethics initiatives with organizational values.*


## Establishing and Leading the Bioethics Committee


- Fletcher, J. C., Boyle, R. J., & Delkeskamp-Hayes, C. (Eds.). (1995). Introduction to Clinical Ethics (2nd ed.). University Publishing Group.
  - *A comprehensive introduction to clinical ethics, offering practical guidance on establishing and leading bioethics committees in healthcare settings.*
- Sugarman, J., & Sulmasy, D. P. (Eds.). (2010). Methods in Medical Ethics (2nd ed.). Georgetown University Press.
  - *Provides an overview of various methodologies used in medical ethics, aiding bioethics program directors in effectively leading ethics committees.*


## Creating a Culture of Ethical Sensitivity and Collaboration


- Gawande, A. (2010). The Checklist Manifesto: How to Get Things Right. Metropolitan Books.
  - *Highlights the importance of checklists in ensuring effective and ethical practices in healthcare, relevant for fostering a culture of ethical sensitivity and collaboration.*

- Roberts, L. W., & Dyer, A. R. (Eds.). (2004). Concise Guide to Ethics in Mental Health Care. American Psychiatric Publishing.
    - *A guide focusing on ethics in mental health care, offering insights into promoting ethical sensitivity and collaborative practices in healthcare settings.*

***

# Chapter 3: Developing a Mission, Vision and Values Statement

Developing Mission, Vision, and Values Statements for a Bioethics Program involves defining the essential components that provide direction, purpose, and ethical grounding. These statements are critical tools that shape the program's activities and ensure alignment with core ethical principles. Crafting them with clarity and precision is vital, whether starting a new Bioethics Program or enhancing an existing one. This process integrates the foundational bioethical principles necessary for establishing a program that is both effective and ethically sound.

## The Role of Mission, Vision, and Values Statements

Mission, Vision, and Values Statements each serve a distinct purpose:

- **Mission Statement**: Defines the program's purpose, primary objectives, and the scope of its activities. It serves as a guide for daily operations and decision-making, ensuring that all actions align with the program's ethical commitments and objectives.
- **Vision Statement:** Articulates the program's long-term goals and aspirations, providing direction for future growth and inspiring both current and future members to work towards a shared objective. It sets a forward-looking goal that aligns with the program's ethical principles and mission.
- **Values Statement**: Outlines the core ethical principles and beliefs that guide the program's actions and decision-making processes. It serves as a moral compass, helping to ensure that the program's activities are consistent with its foundational ethics and are applied in real-world scenarios.

## Developing the Mission Statement

The Mission Statement should succinctly define the purpose and primary objectives of the Bioethics Program. It should clearly state what the program does, why it exists, and who it serves. The following example illustrates a well-aligned Mission Statement for a Bioethics Program:

**Mission Statement**:

The mission of the Bioethics Program is to provide ethics consultation, education, and policy development grounded in the bioethical principles of patient autonomy (informed consent), practitioner beneficence (maximize benefits), practitioner nonmaleficence (minimize burdens), and public justice (ensure fairness). Practitioners are committed to offering treatment options that respect the patient's reasonable goals, values, and priorities while strictly adhering to medical standards of care, institutional policies, and legal mandates. Informed consent is achieved by engaging patients or their legally established surrogates to ensure a clear understanding of their diagnosis, available treatment options (including the option of no treatment), and the potential benefits and risks. When a patient's goals, values, and priorities are unknown, decisions are guided by the principles of nonmaleficence and beneficence within the framework of established medical standards of care. The Bioethics Program is dedicated to fostering ethical awareness, continuous education, and providing leadership in ethical decision-making, ensuring that ethical considerations are integral to all aspects of patient care and organizational policy.

Key Elements:

- Purpose and Objectives: The mission focuses on providing ethics consultation, education, and policy development to support ethical decision-making in healthcare.
- Ethical Foundation: It is rooted in the core bioethical principles of patient autonomy, beneficence, nonmaleficence,

and public justice, ensuring that these principles guide all actions.

- Practitioner and Patient Roles: The statement clarifies that treatment options must align with medical standards, institutional policies, and legal mandates, respecting patient and surrogate involvement in decision-making.
- Informed Consent: It emphasizes the importance of informed consent, ensuring that patients and surrogates understand their medical conditions, options, and associated risks.
- Leadership in Ethics: The statement highlights the program's role in fostering ethical awareness and providing leadership in ethical decision-making.

## Case Study: Crafting a Mission Statement

**Scenario**: A hospital is establishing a new Bioethics Program to support its expanding range of medical services. The Director of the Bioethics Program, Dr. Elaine Martinez, convenes a team of healthcare professionals, including physicians, nurses, and ethics consultants, to develop a Mission Statement. The team's goal is to create a statement that reflects the hospital's commitment to integrating the core bioethical principles—patient autonomy (informed consent), practitioner beneficence (maximize benefits), practitioner nonmaleficence (minimize burdens), and public justice (ensure fairness)—into clinical practice, recognizing that the relative weight of each principle may vary depending on the specific circumstances of each case.

**Approach**: The team conducts a series of workshops to gather input from various departments. They use case studies to discuss real-life ethical dilemmas, focusing on how the Bioethics Program can support the resolution of these dilemmas through a thoughtful and context-sensitive application of bioethical principles. In their discussions, the team emphasizes that while patient autonomy is crucial, it must be balanced with the principles of beneficence, nonmaleficence, and justice, as well as with compliance with medical standards of care, institutional policies, and legal mandates. The team recognizes that, in some situations, one principle may need to take precedence over others to best serve the patient's interests and uphold ethical standards. They also stress the importance of continuous education for healthcare providers to ensure they are equipped to apply these principles effectively.

**Outcome**: The finalized Mission Statement acknowledges the need to specify, weigh, and balance the bioethical principles according to the unique context of each situation. It commits to an ethical decision-making process that considers the patient's reasonable goals, values, and priorities, alongside the need for compliance with established medical standards of care, institutional policies, and legal requirements. This Mission Statement serves as a guiding framework for the Bioethics Program, helping healthcare practitioners navigate complex ethical issues by providing a flexible yet principled approach to ethical decision-making. It reinforces the program's role in ensuring that ethical considerations are central to patient care and that decisions are made with integrity, compassion, and justice.

## Crafting a Vision Statement

A clear and compelling Vision Statement is essential for guiding the development and direction of the Bioethics Program. The Vision Statement should articulate the program's long-term goals and aspirations, reflecting the core values and ethical commitments of the organization. Crafting a Vision Statement involves engaging with stakeholders, including senior leadership, healthcare providers, and patients, to understand their perspectives and priorities. The Vision should be ambitious yet achievable, providing a roadmap for the program's growth and evolution.

**Vision Statement**:

The vision of the Bioethics Program is to create a healthcare environment where ethical principles—patient autonomy (informed consent), practitioner beneficence (maximize benefits), practitioner nonmaleficence (minimize burdens), and public justice (ensure fairness)—are central to all clinical and organizational decisions. By fostering an ethical culture rooted in continuous reflection, dialogue, and education, the program ensures that every decision aligns with medical standards of care, institutional policies, and legal mandates. The Bioethics Program will provide leadership and oversight in ethics consultation and policy development, integrating these principles into both patient care and broader organizational practices. Patient choices will be respected within the boundaries of ethically appropriate treatment options, thereby enhancing the quality, integrity, and compassion of care.

Key Elements:

- Long-term Goals: The vision sets a future where all decisions are guided by the balanced consideration of ethical principles, ensuring thoughtful integration of autonomy, beneficence, nonmaleficence, and justice.
- Ethical Culture: The vision promotes fostering a culture of continuous ethical reflection, dialogue, and collaboration among all healthcare practitioners.
- Integration of Principles: It underscores the importance of specifying, weighing, and balancing bioethical principles within medical standards of care, institutional policies, and legal mandates.
- Leadership and Oversight: The statement emphasizes the program's commitment to providing leadership in ethics consultation and policy development, shaping both patient care and organizational behavior.

**Comprehensive Ethical Engagement**: The vision advocates for thorough patient and surrogate education, ensuring that all parties are equipped to make informed, ethical decisions that align with the patient's reasonable goals, values, and priorities, while also considering the broader ethical implications for society.

## Case Study: Developing a Vision Statement

**Scenario**: The Children's Hospital Ethics Committee is tasked with creating a Vision Statement for its new Bioethics Program. The committee wants to ensure that the Vision Statement reflects the unique needs of pediatric patients, their families, and the healthcare providers caring for them.

**Approach**: The committee holds focus groups with pediatricians, nurses, child psychologists, and patient families. They discuss the ethical challenges specific to pediatric care, such as issues of consent involving minors and parental decision-making. The feedback is used to draft a Vision Statement that emphasizes family-centered care, patient education, and the involvement of children in decision-making processes where appropriate.

**Outcome**: The Vision Statement articulates a future where ethical principles are central to pediatric care, guiding clinical decisions and institutional policies. It inspires healthcare providers to strive for excellence in ethical practice and ensures that the voices of both children and their families are heard and respected in healthcare decisions.

## Involving Stakeholders

Involving stakeholders in the vision-crafting process ensures that the Vision resonates with the broader organization and reflects the collective aspirations of the community. This collaborative approach can help build a sense of ownership and commitment to the Vision, enhancing its impact and sustainability. The director should facilitate discussions, gather input through surveys or focus groups, and synthesize this feedback into a cohesive and inspiring Vision Statement.

Once the Vision is established, it should be communicated consistently and clearly throughout the organization. The director should integrate the Vision into all aspects of the Bioethics Program, from strategic planning and policy development to daily operations and practitioner training. By aligning all activities with the Vision, the director can ensure that the program remains focused and driven toward its long-term goals.

### Regular Review and Adaptation

The Vision Statement should also be periodically reviewed and updated to reflect changes in the organization's priorities, the healthcare landscape, and societal values. This ensures that the Vision remains relevant and continues to inspire and guide the Bioethics Program. Regularly engaging with stakeholders during these reviews can help maintain their commitment and support, ensuring that the Bioethics Program evolves in alignment with its mission and ethical principles.

### Practical Steps for Alignment with Mission and Vision Statements

To ensure that the content of the Bioethics Program aligns with its Mission and Vision Statements, consider the following practical steps:

1. **Patient Autonomy** (Informed Consent):
   - Emphasize the patient's right to informed consent and decision-making based on their reasonable goals, values, and priorities.
   - Ensure patients or surrogates understand their diagnosis, prognosis, available treatment options, the purpose of these options, and the associated benefits and risks.
   - Facilitate logical reasoning and clear communication from patients or surrogates to ensure voluntary and informed consent.
2. **Practitioner Beneficence** (Maximize Benefits):
   - Advocate for maximizing benefits to the patient, aligning actions with the patient's reasonable goals, values, and priorities.
   - Ensure that these actions comply with institutional policies, medical standards of care, and legal requirements.

3. **Practitioner Nonmaleficence** (Minimize Burdens):
   - Focus on avoiding unnecessary harm or risks to the patient.
   - Emphasize minimizing harm while adhering to ethical principles and compliance with institutional policies, medical standards of care, and legal mandates.
4. **Public Justice** (Ensure Fairness):
   - Address fairness and equitable treatment in healthcare decisions, considering the broader implications on society.
   - Ensure adherence to institutional policies, medical standards, and legal frameworks, upholding the principle of public justice.
5. **Compliance Check**:
   - Regularly review content to ensure alignment with bioethical principles and compliance with medical standards, institutional policies, and legal mandates.
   - Promote ethical awareness, understanding, and continuous education among healthcare practitioners and ethics consultants.

## Case Study: Aligning with Mission and Vision

**Scenario**: The Bioethics Program at City General Hospital has received feedback that some healthcare practitioners are unsure how to apply the program's ethical principles in complex cases involving end-of-life care. The Bioethics Director, Dr. James Parker, wants to ensure that the Mission and Vision Statements are effectively guiding clinical practice.

**Approach**: Dr. Parker organizes a series of ethics rounds focusing on end-of-life scenarios. Using the Mission and Vision Statements as a framework, each case is discussed in terms of patient autonomy, beneficence, nonmaleficence, and justice. The rounds are designed to illustrate how these principles can be specified, weighed and balanced in real-life situations, with input from palliative care specialists, nurses, and family members.

**Outcome**: The ethics rounds provide practical examples of how to apply the Mission and Vision Statements. Healthcare practitioners gain confidence in making ethically sound decisions that align with the Bioethics Program's goals. The program's commitment to ethical excellence is reinforced, and patient care is enhanced through better-informed decision-making.

## Integrating TAC with SOAP: Enhancing Ethical Documentation

Combining the Think, Assess, Conclude (TAC) methodology with the SOAP (Subjective, Objective, Assessment, Plan) format enhances the ethical documentation process, making it both comprehensive and aligned with clinical practice standards. This integrated approach ensures that ethical considerations are not only thoroughly analyzed but also clearly communicated within the clinical workflow. By using the widely recognized SOAP format, the Bioethics Program ensures that ethical documentation aligns with healthcare standards, thereby reinforcing the program's mission and vision.

### (S) Subjective: Capturing Perspectives

In the SOAP format, the Subjective section captures the perspectives of patients, surrogates, and healthcare providers. This includes the patient's understanding of their condition, their goals, values, and priorities, and any specific concerns they may have. Documenting these perspectives is crucial for respecting patient autonomy, as it ensures that the patient's voice is central to ethical decision-making. When patients lack decisional capacity, the subjective input should include the surrogate's understanding and representation of the patient's known or reasonably inferred goals, values, and priorities. This section highlights the program's commitment to informed consent and patient-centered care by recording all relevant viewpoints that influence ethical decisions.

### (O) Objective: Providing a Factual Basis

The Objective section records observable and measurable information such as the patient's medical history, current health status, diagnostic results, and other relevant clinical data. Additionally, it should include applicable institutional policies, legal standards, and established medical standards of care. This factual basis is critical for ensuring public justice and practitioner nonmaleficence by providing a clear understanding of the situation and minimizing bias in ethical decision-making. Documenting objective data supports transparency and accountability, ensuring that ethical decisions are grounded in reality and are justifiable.

### (A) Assessment: Ethical Analysis through TAC

In the Assessment section, the TAC methodology is applied to analyze the ethical aspects of the case. This involves:

- **Think**: Identifying the primary ethical issues at stake and the relevant bioethical principles (patient autonomy, beneficence, nonmaleficence, and justice).
- **Assess**: Weighing and balancing these principles in the context of the patient's situation, considering their goals, values, and priorities. The assessment should also consider the broader implications for other patients, healthcare providers, and society, in alignment with public justice.
- **Conclude**: Reaching an ethical conclusion that addresses the identified issues, provides a rationale for the decision, and aligns with medical standards of care, institutional policies, and legal mandates.

This section ensures that ethical reasoning is explicitly documented, making the decision-making process transparent. By integrating TAC into the SOAP format, the assessment becomes a structured ethical reflection, promoting consistency and clarity in clinical ethics consultations.

### (P) Plan: Implementing Ethical Decisions

The Plan section outlines the proposed actions based on the ethical assessment. It should detail:

- **Recommendations and Decisions**: Specific actions to be taken, aligned with the ethical analysis, patient's reasonable goals, values, and priorities, and institutional guidelines.
- **Patient and Surrogate Communication**: Strategies for discussing the ethical decision with the patient or surrogate to ensure understanding and acceptance, reinforcing informed consent.
- **Monitoring and Follow-Up**: Steps for ongoing ethical oversight, including follow-up consultations to reassess the patient's condition and the ethical appropriateness of the plan.

This section translates ethical analysis into actionable steps, ensuring that ethical considerations are operationalized within patient care. By clearly documenting the plan, healthcare providers can ensure adherence to ethical standards and align clinical actions with the Bioethics Program's mission and vision.

## Case Study: Integrating TAC with SOAP

**Scenario**: A patient with advanced Alzheimer's disease is admitted to the hospital with a severe infection. The patient lacks decisional capacity, and their family is divided over whether to pursue aggressive treatment. The ethics consultant, Dr. Karen Lee, is called to facilitate the decision-making process.

**Approach**: Dr. Lee uses the TAC methodology integrated into the SOAP format to document the ethical analysis. In the Subjective section, she captures the perspectives of the family members, the healthcare team, and any previously stated wishes of the patient. The Objective section includes the patient's medical condition, prognosis, and applicable hospital policies. Dr. Lee conducts an ethical assessment by identifying the primary ethical issues, weighing the principles of beneficence, nonmaleficence, and patient autonomy as interpreted by the family. She concludes with a recommendation that balances these principles, suggesting a treatment plan that aligns with the patient's values and the family's consensus.

**Outcome**: The integrated TAC methodology and SOAP Notes documentation provides a clear, structured record of the ethical decision-making process. The family feels supported, and the healthcare team has a clear plan of action. The case demonstrates how the Bioethics Program's mission and vision are applied in practice, ensuring that ethical considerations are at the forefront of patient care.

## Setting Short-term and Long-term Goals

Setting well-defined goals is vital for translating the Bioethics Program's vision into concrete actions. Short-term goals focus on immediate improvements, while long-term goals aim to establish sustained impact and growth, all while adhering to the core bioethical principles of patient autonomy, beneficence, nonmaleficence, and justice.

### Short-Term Goals Examples:

1. **Establish an Ethics Consultation Process**:
   - Goal: Develop and implement a standardized ethics consultation process within the first six months.
   - Action Steps: Design consultation guidelines that incorporate Think, Assess and Conclude (TAC) methodology and SOAP Notes documentation, and pilot the process in a selected department.
   - Alignment with Vision: A structured consultation process promotes consistent ethical decision-making, ensuring that all cases are evaluated using a standardized approach aligned with bioethical principles.
2. **Conduct Ethics Education Workshops**:
   - Goal: Organize quarterly workshops focused on key ethical issues, case studies, and the integration of the Think, Assess,

and Conclude (TAC) methodology and SOAP Notes documentation.

- Action Steps: Develop workshop content, schedule sessions, and engage experts to lead discussions.
- Alignment with Vision: These workshops will enhance ethical competence among healthcare providers, fostering an ethical culture and aligning clinical practices with the program's vision.

3. **Develop an Ethics Consultation Handbook**:
   - Goal: Create and distribute a handbook detailing the ethics consultation process, including the use of The Think, Assess, and Conclude (TAC) methodology and SOAP Notes documentation.
   - Action Steps: Draft handbook content, review for accuracy and comprehensiveness, and ensure distribution to all relevant departments.
   - Alignment with Vision: The handbook serves as a reference tool, supporting consistent and informed ethical decision-making across the institution.
4. **Launch a Bioethics Program Awareness Campaign**:
   - Goal: Increase program visibility and understanding among healthcare practitioners within four months.
   - Action Steps: Develop promotional materials, organize informational sessions, and create a dedicated intranet page.
   - Alignment with Vision: Raising awareness ensures that practitioners know how to access ethical resources, promoting an ethical culture institution-wide.
5. **Initiate Monthly Ethics Rounds**:
   - Goal: Start monthly interdisciplinary ethics rounds to discuss real cases and ethical challenges.

- Action Steps: Plan and schedule rounds, prepare case studies, and facilitate discussions using The Think, Assess, and Conclude (TAC) methodology and SOAP Notes documentation frameworks.
- Alignment with Vision: Regular ethics rounds promote continuous learning and ethical dialogue, integral to the program's vision of an ethical culture.

**Long-Term Goals Examples:**

1. **Expand Ethics Consultation Services**:
    - Goal: Extend consultation services to all clinical departments within three years.
    - Action Steps: Develop tailored protocols, recruit additional consultants, and implement a tracking system for consultations.
    - Strategic Alignment: Expanding services ensures comprehensive ethical support, aligning with the program's vision of integrating ethical considerations across the institution.
2. **Develop a Comprehensive Ethics Education Curriculum**:
    - Goal: Establish a robust curriculum for all healthcare practitioners within five years.
    - Action Steps: Collaborate with academic partners, develop accredited courses, and implement online learning platforms.
    - Strategic Alignment: A comprehensive education program supports lifelong learning and ethical excellence, equipping practitioners with the skills to navigate ethical challenges.
3. **Create a Center for Bioethics Research and Innovation**:
    - Goal: Establish a dedicated bioethics research center within five to seven years.
    - Action Steps: Secure funding, recruit bioethics experts, and initiate interdisciplinary research projects.

- Strategic Alignment: The research center will advance bioethics knowledge and position the institution as a leader in ethical healthcare practices.

4. **Enhance Engagement with the Bioethics Community**:
   - Goal: Strengthen partnerships with bioethics organizations within five years.
   - Action Steps: Host conferences, participate in joint research, and contribute to policy development.
   - Strategic Alignment: Engagement with the bioethics community ensures that the program stays informed about ethical advancements and contributes to broader ethical discussions.
5. **Implement a System-Wide Ethics Policy Framework**:
   - Goal: Develop a standardized ethics policy framework across the healthcare system within four years.
   - Action Steps: Review existing policies, develop new guidelines, and train staff on the new framework.
   - Strategic Alignment: A consistent policy framework ensures that all practices are guided by ethical principles, reinforcing the program's vision.
6. **Foster Interdisciplinary Collaboration**:
   - Goal: Integrate bioethics into all clinical and research initiatives within three years.
   - Action Steps: Form interdisciplinary ethics committees, include ethics in research protocols, and hold regular discussion forums.
   - Strategic Alignment: Interdisciplinary collaboration strengthens the ethical culture, ensuring that ethical considerations are integral to all healthcare activities.

## Case Study: Setting Goals

**Scenario**: The Bioethics Program at Regional Medical Center is looking to expand its services to cover more departments. The program director, Dr. Lisa Carter, wants to set both short-term and long-term goals to guide this expansion.

**Approach**: Dr. Carter conducts a needs assessment across various departments to identify areas requiring immediate ethical support. Based on this assessment, she sets short-term goals to establish ethics consultation processes in the emergency and intensive care units within the first six months. For long-term goals, Dr. Carter aims to expand ethics consultation services to all clinical departments over three years, recruit additional ethics consultants, and implement training programs.

**Outcome**: By setting clear, realistic goals, the Bioethics Program can strategically expand its services. Short-term goals provide immediate improvements, while long-term goals ensure sustainable growth. The alignment with the program's mission and vision is maintained throughout the process, enhancing ethical support across the institution.

## Resource Considerations

In setting both short-term and long-term goals, the director should consider the resources and capabilities of the organization. This involves conducting a thorough assessment of the current state of the Bioethics Program, identifying strengths and areas for improvement, and determining the resources needed to achieve the goals. By aligning goals with available resources, the director can ensure that the Bioethics Program is both ambitious and realistic.

**Resource Considerations Examples:**

**1. Assessment of Current Staffing Levels:**

- Scenario: Before expanding the scope of ethics consultations, the director conducts a staffing assessment and discovers that the current team is already operating at full capacity.

- Resource Consideration: The director decides to prioritize the recruitment and training of additional ethics consultants before implementing the expansion plan. This ensures that the program can meet the increased demand for consultations without overburdening the existing team.
- Outcome: By aligning the expansion goal with available staffing resources, the program is able to scale its services sustainably. This approach maintains the quality of consultations, avoids burnout among staff, and ensures that ethical principles, such as practitioner nonmaleficence (minimize burdens) to both patients and staff, are upheld.

2. **Budget Allocation for Ethics Education**:
   - Scenario: The program has a limited budget for the upcoming fiscal year, but there is a high demand for ethics education workshops.
   - Resource Consideration: The director opts to focus on developing online learning modules as a cost-effective alternative to in-person workshops. This approach allows the program to reach a larger audience while staying within budget constraints.
   - Outcome: By choosing online modules, the program meets the educational needs of healthcare providers without exceeding financial limits. This decision aligns with the principles of beneficence (maximize benefits) by providing valuable education and public justice (ensure fairness) by making ethics education accessible to more practitioners.
3. **Technology Infrastructure for Digital Tools**:
   - Scenario: The program aims to enhance communication by leveraging digital tools, such as creating a dedicated website and social media presence. However, the current IT infrastructure is outdated and may not support these initiatives effectively.

- Resource Consideration: The director collaborates with the IT department to upgrade the necessary technology infrastructure before launching the digital tools. This may involve reallocating funds from less critical projects or seeking additional funding through grants.
- Outcome: Ensuring a robust technology infrastructure supports the ethical principle of justice by providing equitable access to resources. It also aligns with the program's commitment to patient autonomy by enhancing communication pathways, thereby facilitating informed decision-making.

4. **Physical Space for Ethics Consultations**:
   - Scenario: The program plans to increase the number of in-person ethics consultations, but the current office space is limited and does not accommodate private discussions comfortably.
   - Resource Consideration: The director identifies the need for additional private meeting rooms and collaborates with the facility management team to reallocate space within the institution. If additional space cannot be immediately secured, temporary solutions, such as booking external conference rooms or using virtual consultations, are considered.
   - Outcome: By ensuring private and comfortable consultation settings, the program upholds the principles of autonomy and confidentiality, essential for effective ethics consultations. This also aligns with the ethical commitment to provide a safe environment for sensitive discussions, reflecting nonmaleficence (minimize burdens).
5. **Financial Planning for Long-term Initiatives**:
   - Scenario: The program aims to establish a Center for Bioethics Research and Innovation over the next five years. However, the initial cost estimates exceed the current financial resources available to the program.

- Resource Consideration: The director decides to break the project into phases, starting with smaller, fundable initiatives such as securing seed funding, building partnerships, and conducting preliminary research. This phased approach allows the program to gradually build toward the larger goal while managing financial risks.
- Outcome: By aligning the long-term goal with realistic financial planning, the program makes steady progress toward establishing the research center. This phased approach supports the principle of beneficence by gradually increasing the program's capacity to contribute positively to bioethics research without compromising its financial stability.

6. **Leveraging Existing Expertise within the Institution**:
   - Scenario: The program plans to develop a comprehensive ethics policy framework but lacks in-house legal expertise to navigate the complex regulatory landscape.
   - Resource Consideration: The director leverages existing resources by partnering with the institution's legal department and external legal experts to provide guidance and support. This collaboration ensures that the policy framework is both comprehensive and compliant with legal standards.
   - Outcome: Utilizing existing expertise promotes efficiency and reduces costs while ensuring that policies are legally sound and ethically robust. This approach supports public justice by ensuring that all policies adhere to legal requirements, thereby protecting patient rights and maintaining public trust.

## Developing the Values Statement

A Values Statement articulates the core ethical principles that guide the Bioethics Program's actions and decision-making processes. It reinforces the importance of these principles in every aspect of the program's work and emphasizes their practical implementation. Below is an example of a Values Statement for a Bioethics Program:

### Values Statement:

The values of the Bioethics Program are grounded in the principles of patient autonomy (informed consent), practitioner beneficence (maximize benefits), practitioner nonmaleficence (minimize burdens), and public justice (ensure fairness). These principles are specified, weighed, and balanced according to the unique context of each case, ensuring alignment with established medical standards of care, institutional policies, and legal mandates. The program is committed to embedding these values into all aspects of patient care and decision-making, providing leadership in ethical practice, and fostering an environment where ethical considerations are a fundamental part of both clinical practice and organizational behavior.

Key Elements:

- Ethical Principles: The values statement clearly identifies the core bioethical principles guiding the program.
- Contextual Application: It acknowledges that these principles must be specified, weighed, and balanced in each unique context, adhering to medical standards, policies, and legal requirements.
- Commitment to Practice: The statement emphasizes the practical application of these values, ensuring they actively shape patient care, decision-making, and organizational behavior.
- Leadership in Ethics: It highlights the program's commitment to providing ethical leadership and fostering an environment where ethical considerations are integral to healthcare.

## Communicating the Mission, Vision, and Values to Stakeholders

Effective communication is essential for gaining buy-in and support for the Bioethics Program's Mission, Vision, and Values. The director should use a variety of communication channels to share these statements with stakeholders and engage them in the program's goals.

**Tailored Communication**:

- Audience-specific Messaging: Clear and consistent communication helps ensure that all stakeholders understand and support the program's goals. The director should tailor messages to different audiences, emphasizing aspects most relevant to each group. For example, senior leadership may be interested in how the program aligns with organizational goals, while clinical practitioners may focus on how it supports patient care and professional development.
- Engagement Strategies: Engage stakeholders through regular meetings, newsletters, presentations, and interactive sessions. Providing opportunities for feedback and involvement fosters a sense of ownership and commitment, enhancing the program's success and sustainability.

**Ongoing Engagement**:

- Continuous Reinforcement: Communication should not be limited to initial announcements. The director should ensure that communication efforts are ongoing, regularly revisiting and reinforcing the Mission, Vision, and Values through various channels. This continuous engagement helps maintain momentum and ensures that the Bioethics Program remains aligned with the evolving needs and priorities of the organization and its stakeholders.

Expanding Communication Beyond Internal Stakeholders:

- External Engagement: Communication should also extend beyond internal stakeholders to include external partners and the broader community. This can involve presenting the Bioethics Program's Mission, Vision, and Values at conferences, publishing articles in academic journals, and engaging with media to raise awareness about the program's work.

- Visibility and Collaboration: By promoting the Bioethics Program's achievements and initiatives, the director can enhance its visibility and reputation, attracting support and collaboration from a wider audience.

**Leveraging Digital Tools**:

- Digital Presence: In addition to traditional communication channels, the director should leverage digital tools and platforms to reach a broader audience. This can include creating a dedicated website or social media presence for the Bioethics Program, where updates, resources, and educational materials can be shared.
- Interactive Engagement: By utilizing digital communication strategies, the director can engage with stakeholders in a more dynamic and interactive way, fostering a sense of community and collaboration.

**Conclusion**

By integrating these elements into the Bioethics Program's strategic planning, the program can ensure that its Mission, Vision, and Values are not only communicated effectively but also implemented consistently across all levels of the organization. This comprehensive approach supports the program's commitment to ethical excellence, aligning all activities with the foundational bioethical principles of patient autonomy, beneficence, nonmaleficence, and public justice. It ensures that the Bioethics Program remains a vital and integral part of patient care, practitioner support, and the broader healthcare community.

***

The following templates are designed to help the Bioethics Program Director and team systematically develop, review, and communicate their Mission, Vision, and Values, ensuring these foundational elements are effectively integrated into the program and aligned with the broader organizational goals.

***

## 3.1 Mission Statement Development Template

**Purpose**: To guide the development of a clear and concise Mission Statement for the Bioethics Program.

**Date**: [Date]
**Prepared by**: [Name]

**Purpose of the Bioethics Program**

- What is the primary purpose of the Bioethics Program?
  [Insert Purpose Statement]

**Primary Objectives**

- What are the key objectives of the program?
  [List Key Objectives]

**Scope of Activities**

- What specific activities will the program engage in? (e.g., ethics consultations, education, policy development)
  [List Activities]

**Ethical Foundation**

- Which core bioethical principles will guide the program?
  [List Principles: Patient Autonomy, Practitioner Beneficence, Practitioner Nonmaleficence, Public Justice]

**Practitioner and Patient Roles**

- How will the roles and responsibilities of practitioners and patients be defined within the program?
  [Describe Roles and Responsibilities]

**Educational Commitment**

- How will the program foster ethical awareness and understanding among healthcare practitioners?
  [Describe Educational Initiatives]

**Draft Mission Statement**

- [Combine the elements above into a succinct Mission Statement]

**Review and Approval**

- Has the Mission Statement been reviewed by key stakeholders?

  ☐ Yes

  ☐ No

**Date of Final Approval**: [Date]
**Approved by:** [Name/Title]

***

## 3.2 Vision Statement Development Template

**Purpose**: To outline the long-term goals and aspirations of the Bioethics Program, ensuring alignment with the organization's ethical commitments.

**Date**: [Date]
**Prepared by**: [Name]

**Long-term Goals**

- What are the program's long-term aspirations?
  [List Long-term Goals]

**Ethical Culture**

- How does the program aim to influence the broader ethical culture within the institution?
  [Describe Cultural Impact]

**Integration of Principles**

- How will the four core bioethical principles be integrated into clinical decisions and organizational practices?
  [Describe Integration Strategy]

**Stakeholder Engagement**

- How will stakeholders be involved in the vision development process?
  [Describe Engagement Process]

**Draft Vision Statement**

[Combine the elements above into a cohesive Vision Statement]

**Review and Approval**

- Has the Vision Statement been reviewed by key stakeholders?
  ☐ Yes
  ☐ No

**Date of Final Approval**: [Date]
**Approved by**: [Name/Title]

***

## 3.3 Values Statement Development Template

**Purpose**: To articulate the core ethical principles that will guide the Bioethics Program's actions and decision-making processes.

**Date**: [Date]
**Prepared by**: [Name]

**Core Ethical Principles**

- What are the fundamental bioethical principles that guide the program?
  [List Principles: Patient Autonomy, Practitioner Beneficence, Practitioner Nonmaleficence, Public Justice]

**Contextual Application**

- How will these principles be specified and balanced within the context of medical standards of care, institutional policies, and legal requirements?
  [Describe Contextual Application]

**Commitment to Practice**

- How will the program ensure these values are implemented in practice?
  [Describe Practical Implementation]

**Draft Values Statement**

- [Combine the elements above into a coherent Values Statement]

**Review and Approval**

- Has the Values Statement been reviewed by key stakeholders?
  ☐ Yes
  ☐ No

**Date of Final Approval**: [Date]
**Approved by**: [Name/Title]

***

## 3.4 Communication Plan Template

**Purpose**: To create a structured plan for communicating the Mission, Vision, and Values of the Bioethics Program to stakeholders.

**Date**: [Date]
**Prepared by**: [Name]

**Target Audience**

- Who are the primary stakeholders for the Bioethics Program?
  [List Stakeholders: e.g., senior leadership, clinical staff, patients]

**Key Messages**

- What are the key messages to communicate?
  [List Key Messages: e.g., the importance of the Mission, Vision, and Values]

**Communication Channels**

- Through which channels will the Mission, Vision, and Values be communicated?
  [List Channels: e.g., meetings, newsletters, presentations, social media]

**Timeline**

- What is the timeline for communication activities?
  [Provide Timeline: e.g., initial launch, regular updates]

**Engagement Strategies**

- How will you ensure ongoing engagement with the Mission, Vision, and Values?
  [Describe Strategies: e.g., regular meetings, feedback mechanisms]

**Review and Feedback**

- How will the effectiveness of the communication be assessed? [Describe Review Process: e.g., surveys, interviews, feedback forms]

**Implementation Steps**

[List steps required to implement the communication plan]

**Approval and Review**

- Has the Communication Plan been reviewed by key stakeholders?
  ☐ Yes
  ☐ No

**Date of Final Approval**: [Date]
**Approved by**: [Name/Title]

***

# Further Readings and References


## Crafting a Vision Statement

- Collins, J. C., & Porras, J. I. (1994). Built to Last: Successful Habits of Visionary Companies. Harper Business.
  - *Explores the characteristics of visionary companies and the importance of crafting enduring vision statements, providing guidance for bioethics program directors.*
- Kouzes, J. M., & Posner, B. Z. (2017). The Leadership Challenge: How to Make Extraordinary Things Happen in Organizations (6th ed.). Wiley.
  - *Offers practical advice on leadership and the creation of compelling vision statements, relevant for bioethics program directors.*

## Setting Short-term and Long-term Goals

- Doran, G. T. (1981). There's a S.M.A.R.T. way to write management's goals and objectives. Management Review, 70(11), 35-36.
  - *Introduces the S.M.A.R.T. criteria for setting effective goals, providing a structured approach for bioethics program directors to develop short-term and long-term goals.*
- Covey, S. R. (1989). The 7 Habits of Highly Effective People: Powerful Lessons in Personal Change. Simon & Schuster.
  - *Discusses the principles of personal and organizational effectiveness, offering insights into goal-setting and achieving long-term success.*

## Communicating Your Vision and Mission to Stakeholders

- Kotter, J. P. (2012). Leading Change. Harvard Business Review Press.
  - *Examines the process of leading organizational change and effectively communicating vision and mission statements to stakeholders.*

- Sinek, S. (2009). Start with Why: How Great Leaders Inspire Everyone to Take Action. Penguin Group.
    - *Emphasizes the importance of understanding and communicating the underlying purpose (the "Why") behind an organization's vision and mission.*

***

# Review Questions

**True/False Questions:**

1. The foundational principles of bioethics include patient autonomy, practitioner beneficence, practitioner nonmaleficence, and public justice.
True or False?

2. The role of a Bioethics Program Director includes updating knowledge of emerging ethical issues.
True or False?

3. Establishing a culture of ethical awareness within an organization involves integrating bioethical principles into everyday practice.
True or False?

4. Preventive ethics activities are not a significant part of a Bioethics Program Director's responsibilities.
True or False?

5. The Mission Statement should primarily focus on the long-term goals of the Bioethics Program.
True or False?

**Multiple-Choice Questions:**

6. What is a crucial component of a Bioethics Program Director's role in fostering ethical sensitivity?
a) Ignoring practitioners concerns about ethical issues
b) Conducting regular ethics rounds and workshops
c) Avoiding interdisciplinary collaboration
d) Focusing solely on clinical practices

7. Which principle is NOT one of the four foundational principles of bioethics?
a) Patient autonomy
b) Practitioner beneficence
c) Public justice
d) Financial efficiency

**Clinical Vignettes:**

8. A hospital has recently introduced genetic testing for personalized medicine. A patient expresses concern about privacy and potential discrimination. What is the best course of action for the Bioethics Program Director?
a) Dismiss the patient's concerns as unfounded
b) Explain the ethical implications and privacy measures in place
c) Suggest the patient avoid genetic testing altogether
d) Recommend the patient consult a lawyer

9. During an ethics consultation, a conflict arises between a patient's family and the healthcare team regarding end-of-life care decisions. What should the Bioethics Program Director do?
a) Side with the healthcare team
b) Facilitate a meeting to mediate the discussion and find common ground
c) Ignore the conflict
d) Advise the family to seek another healthcare provider

10. A healthcare provider raises an ethical concern about the allocation of limited resources during a crisis. What is the best approach for the Bioethics Program Director?
a) Dismiss the concern as irrelevant
b) Review the current policies and ensure they are ethically sound and fair
c) Tell the provider to follow orders without question
d) Avoid addressing the issue until after the crisis

## Correct Answers:

1. True
2. True
3. True
4. False (Preventive ethics activities are a significant part of a Bioethics Program Director's responsibilities.)
5. False (The Mission Statement should primarily focus on the purpose, primary objectives, and daily operations of the Bioethics Program, not the long-term goals. The long-term goals are typically addressed in the Vision Statement.)
6. b) Conducting regular ethics rounds and workshops
7. d) Financial efficiency
8. b) Explain the ethical implications and privacy measures in place
9. b) Facilitate a meeting to mediate the discussion and find common ground
10. b) Review the current policies and ensure they are ethically sound and fair

***

# Part II: Core Responsibilities of a Bioethics Program Director

## Chapter 4: Conducting Healthcare Ethics Consultations

### Overview of Healthcare Ethics Consultations

Healthcare ethics consultations are a structured and systematic process for addressing ethical issues that arise in clinical practice. These consultations are critical in guiding ethical decision-making by incorporating the perspectives of patients, families, and healthcare providers. The primary goal is to facilitate informed and ethically sound decision-making, ensuring that the values and preferences of all parties involved are respected and that decisions align with bioethical principles, such as patient autonomy (informed consent), practitioner beneficence (maximize benefits), practitioner nonmaleficence (minimize burdens), and public justice (ensure fairness).

As the Bioethics Program Director, your role includes ensuring that ethics consultations are conducted effectively, with a strong emphasis on clarity, transparency, and empathy. This involves establishing and adhering to clear protocols that guide the initiation, execution, and documentation of consultations. Effective consultations rely on gathering comprehensive and relevant information, understanding the context, and fostering an open dialogue among all parties involved. This process helps to streamline the ethical analysis and ensures that decisions are well-informed and ethically justified.

Ethics consultations often involve complex and sensitive issues, such as end-of-life care decisions, conflicts between patients and healthcare providers, and challenges related to informed consent.

Addressing these issues requires a nuanced understanding of the ethical principles at stake and the ability to mediate between conflicting values or interests. The director must ensure that consultations are handled with the utmost care and professionalism, maintaining the integrity of the ethical analysis and respecting the dignity and autonomy of all individuals involved.

## Establishing Clear Protocols

To facilitate effective consultations, the Bioethics Program Director should establish clear protocols that guide the process. These protocols should outline:

1. **Initiation of Consultations**: Clearly define the circumstances under which a consultation can be requested, who can request it, and the process for initiating a consultation. This ensures that ethical issues are identified and addressed promptly.
2. **Conducting Consultations**: Define the steps involved in conducting the consultation, including gathering relevant information, interviewing stakeholders, and consulting ethical guidelines and legal standards. The consultation process should be structured to ensure that all perspectives are considered and that the ethical analysis is comprehensive.
3. **Documentation and Communication**: Establish guidelines for documenting the consultation process, including the ethical issues identified, the analysis conducted, and the recommendations made. Documentation should be clear, concise, and accessible, providing a record for future reference and ensuring accountability.
4. **Follow-Up**: Implement a follow-up process to monitor the outcomes of the consultation, ensure that recommendations are implemented, and address any ongoing ethical concerns. Follow-up is essential for evaluating the effectiveness of the consultation and ensuring continuous improvement.

## Addressing Systemic Issues

In addition to addressing individual cases, the Bioethics Program Director should take a proactive approach to identifying and addressing systemic issues that may give rise to ethical dilemmas. This can involve:

- Analyzing Trends in Consultation Data: Regularly review consultation data to identify patterns or recurring issues. Understanding these trends can help pinpoint underlying causes of ethical conflicts and inform the development of preventive measures.
- Implementing Preventive Measures: Develop strategies to address systemic issues, such as enhancing communication channels, clarifying institutional policies, or addressing conflicts of interest. By proactively addressing these issues, the director can reduce the likelihood of ethical dilemmas arising and improve the overall ethical climate of the organization.
- Promoting Ethical Awareness and Education: Educate healthcare practitioners about common ethical issues and the importance of ethical decision-making. Providing training on ethical principles, decision-making frameworks, and consultation procedures equips practitioners with the skills and knowledge needed to handle ethical dilemmas confidently and competently.

## Interprofessional Collaboration

Effective ethics consultations require input from a range of stakeholders, including physicians, nurses, social workers, legal experts, and others. As the Bioethics Program Director, it is essential to facilitate collaboration among these stakeholders to ensure a holistic and comprehensive approach to ethical decision-making. Interprofessional collaboration enriches the ethical analysis by incorporating diverse perspectives and expertise, leading to more balanced and well-rounded decisions.

## Case Study 1: End-of-Life Decision-Making in a Interprofessional Context

**Scenario**: A patient with advanced cancer is admitted to the ICU with severe respiratory distress. The patient has a Do Not Resuscitate (DNR) order, but the family requests all possible measures to prolong life, including intubation. The ICU team is conflicted, wanting to respect the patient's wishes but also considering the family's distress.

**Consultation Process**:

1. **Initiation**: The ICU team requests an ethics consultation to navigate the conflict between the patient's documented wishes and the family's requests.
2. **Information Gathering**: The ethics consultant reviews the patient's medical records, including the DNR order, and meets with the ICU team, the patient's family, and other relevant stakeholders.
3. **Ethical Analysis**: Using the Think, Assess, and Conclude (TAC) methodology, the ethics consultant analyzes the ethical principles involved, emphasizing patient autonomy (the DNR order), practitioner nonmaleficence (minimize burdens by not providing futile treatment), and public justice (fair allocation of medical resources).
4. **Recommendation**: The ethics consultant recommends honoring the patient's DNR order while providing palliative care to ensure comfort. The consultant also suggests involving a palliative care specialist to support the family and address their concerns.

**Outcome**: The patient's autonomy is respected, and the family receives support, aligning with ethical principles and enhancing the quality of care.

## Training and Education

Training practitioners in effective consultation techniques is crucial for ensuring consistency and quality in ethics consultations. The Bioethics Program Director should develop and implement training programs that cover:

- **Ethical Analysis**: Teaching practitioners how to identify ethical issues, apply ethical principles, and use decision-making frameworks like the Think, Assess, and Conclude (TAC) methodology.
- **Communication Skills**: Training on how to conduct sensitive conversations, listen actively, and facilitate open discussions among stakeholders.
- **Conflict Resolution**: Equipping practitioners with skills to manage conflicts and navigate disagreements effectively.

## Monitoring and Evaluation

To ensure the effectiveness of ethics consultations, the Bioethics Program Director should establish a system for monitoring and evaluating consultations. This can include:

- **Feedback from Participants**: Gathering feedback from patients, families, and healthcare providers involved in consultations to assess the consultation's impact and identify areas for improvement.
- **Review of Consultation Outcomes**: Regularly reviewing the outcomes of consultations to determine whether recommendations were implemented and whether they achieved the desired ethical outcomes.
- **Periodic Audits**: Conducting audits of consultation practices and documentation to ensure compliance with established protocols and ethical standards.

### Case Study 2: Informed Consent in Complex Medical Cases

**Scenario**: A patient with a chronic neurological condition is offered a new, experimental treatment. The treatment has potential benefits but also significant risks. The patient is eager to proceed, but their family expresses concerns about the risks and potential impact on the patient's quality of life.

### Consultation Process:

1. **Initiation**: The treating practitioner requests an ethics consultation to ensure the patient's decision is fully informed and ethically sound.
2. **Information Gathering**: The ethics consultant reviews the patient's medical history, the qualifications of the practitioner conducting the research, details of the experimental treatment, and the Institutional Review Board (IRB) approval documentation, and also meets with the patient and their family.
3. **Ethical Analysis**: Using Think, Assess and Conclude (TAC) methodology, the ethics consultant determines if the practitioner has IRB approval, and if so, then evaluates the patient's autonomy (desire to proceed), practitioner beneficence (potential benefits of the treatment), practitioner nonmaleficence (risks involved), and public justice (fairness in accessing experimental treatments).
4. **Recommendation**: The ethics consultant recommends providing the patient and family with comprehensive information about the treatment, including potential outcomes, risks, and alternatives. A decision-making aid is provided to help the patient and family make an informed choice.

**Outcome**: The patient and family are able to make a well-informed decision, aligning with ethical principles and respecting the patient's autonomy.

## Integrating Ethics Consultations into Quality Improvement

Ethics consultations should be integrated into the overall quality improvement initiatives of the organization. This integration can enhance patient care, improve communication, and reduce conflicts by ensuring that ethical considerations are embedded in all aspects of clinical practice. The Bioethics Program Director should work to align ethics consultation practices with broader organizational goals and quality improvement efforts.

## Encouraging Peer Support and Mentoring

In addition to formal training and evaluation, the Bioethics Program Director should encourage informal peer support and mentoring among practitioners. This can involve creating opportunities for practitioners to discuss their experiences with ethical dilemmas and learn from each other. Peer support helps build a community of practice, fostering ethical awareness and shared learning.

## Conclusion

Conducting healthcare ethics consultations is a fundamental responsibility of the Bioethics Program Director. By establishing clear protocols, promoting interprofessional collaboration, providing training and education, and integrating ethics consultations into quality improvement efforts, the director can ensure that ethical decision-making is a core component of patient care. Real-world case studies and examples further enhance the understanding and application of ethical principles, ensuring that the Bioethics Program remains responsive to the needs of patients, families, and healthcare providers.

***

The following structured processes, forms, and templates offer a robust framework for conducting effective ethics consultations within the Bioethics Program. These tools are designed to ensure that each consultation is thorough, respectful of all perspectives, and grounded in ethical and legal standards. By following these guidelines, healthcare professionals can navigate complex ethical dilemmas with clarity and empathy, promoting high-quality patient care and fostering a culture of ethical excellence within the organization.

***

## 4.1 Structured Process for Ethics Consultations

**Purpose**: To provide a comprehensive and systematic framework for conducting healthcare ethics consultations with clarity, transparency, and empathy, while promoting continuous improvement and ethical excellence.

### — I. Initiating an Ethics Consultation

1. **Request Submission**:
   - Any practitioner, patient, or family member can initiate a consultation.
   - Requests should be submitted through a standardized form available in both physical and digital formats.
2. **Initial Review**:
   - The Bioethics Program Director or designated ethics consultant reviews the request to determine urgency and appropriateness.
   - Immediate consultations are prioritized if the situation involves urgent clinical decisions, such as end-of-life care.

---

### — II. Gathering Information

1. **Medical Records Review**:
   - Collect all relevant medical records, including patient history, current treatment plans, and previous consultations.
2. **Stakeholder Interviews**:
   - Conduct interviews with key stakeholders, including the patient (if possible), family members, attending physicians, nurses, and any other relevant healthcare providers.
   - Ensure that all perspectives are documented and considered.
3. **Ethical and Legal Guidelines**:
   - Review pertinent ethical guidelines and legal standards relevant to the case.
   - Consult institutional policies and professional guidelines from recognized bodies like the American Medical Association (AMA) or the American Society for Bioethics

and Humanities (ASBH).

---

## — III. Conducting the Consultation

1. **Interprofessional Team Meeting**:
    - Assemble a interprofessional team, including physicians, nurses, social workers, legal experts, and ethicists.
    - Facilitate a structured discussion, ensuring that all voices are heard and respected.
2. **Ethical Analysis**:
    - Use ethical decision-making frameworks (e.g., the Four Principles Approach: autonomy, beneficence, nonmaleficence, justice).
    - Systematically analyze the ethical dimensions of the case, considering the values and preferences of all parties involved.
3. **Documentation**:
    - Document the consultation process, including the ethical analysis, discussions, and final recommendations.
    - Ensure that the documentation is clear, comprehensive, and accessible for future reference.

---

## — IV. Providing Support

1. **Communication**:
    - Communicate findings and recommendations to all stakeholders in a clear and empathetic manner.
    - Offer to facilitate discussions between conflicting parties to achieve a resolution.
2. **Emotional Support**:
    - Provide emotional support to patients, families, and healthcare providers affected by the ethical dilemma.
    - Consider involving chaplaincy services or professional counselors if needed.

---

## — V. Monitoring and Evaluation

1. **Feedback Mechanisms**:
   - Gather feedback from participants after each consultation to assess the process and outcomes.
   - Use feedback to identify areas for improvement.
2. **Periodic Audits**:
   - Conduct regular audits of the consultation process to ensure consistency and quality.
   - Review consultation outcomes to measure effectiveness and adherence to ethical standards.
3. **Continuous Improvement**:
   - Implement continuous improvement efforts based on feedback and audit results.
   - Promote ongoing learning and development to maintain high standards of ethical practice.

---

## — VI. Addressing Systemic Issues

1. **Data Analysis**:
   - Regularly analyze consultation data to identify trends and recurring ethical issues.
   - Use this data to inform organizational policies and practices.
2. **Preventive Measures**:
   - Implement preventive measures to address underlying causes of ethical dilemmas.
   - Develop and refine institutional policies to mitigate common ethical conflicts.

By following this structured process, healthcare ethics consultations can be conducted effectively, ensuring clarity, transparency, and empathy while addressing both individual cases and systemic ethical issues. This comprehensive approach will help maintain high standards of ethical practice and promote a culture of continuous improvement and ethical excellence within the organization.

***

## 4.2 TAC Methodology & SOAP Documentation

**Purpose**: To provide a structured framework for ethical consultation and decision-making, focusing on the bioethical principles of Patient Autonomy, Practitioner Beneficence, Practitioner Nonmaleficence, and Public Justice.

**Patient Name**: ______________________________
**Date of Birth**: ______________________________
**Medical Record Number**: ______________________
**Primary Diagnosis**: __________________________
**Current Treatment Plan**: ______________________

---

### (T) THINK

- **Ethical Dilemma**: Articulate the ethical dilemma or topic clearly.
- **Case Details**: Gather and review case details, including medical history and patient circumstances.
- **Boundaries**: Ensure a thorough understanding of medical standards of care, institutional policies, and legal mandates and prohibitions.
- **Stakeholders**: Identify all individuals and entities impacted by the ethical issue (e.g., patient, family, healthcare team, institution, community). Consider broader impacts, such as societal or public health implications, if relevant.

## (A) ASSESS

1. **Patient Autonomy** (Informed Consent):
    - **Specification**: Practitioner has determined that the patient or surrogate has provided informed consent.
    - **Informed Consent's Necessary Conditions:**
      (all boxes must be checked for informed consent)
      - [ ] **Decisional Capacity**: The patient or surrogate has the ability to understand and make informed decisions about their care.
      - [ ] **Diagnosis and Prognosis**: The patient or surrogate understands their medical condition and the likely outcomes.
      - [ ] **Treatment Options**: All available treatment options (including no treatment) that comply with medical standards of care, institutional policies, and legal mandates and prohibitions have been presented.
      - [ ] **Benefits and Risks**: The patient or surrogate understands the benefits and risks associated with each treatment option.
      - [ ] **Coercion**: The patient or surrogate is making a voluntary choice free from pressure or coercion; practitioners should assess and document any signs or sources of coercion.
      - [ ] **Goals, Values, and Priorities**: The treatment decision aligns with the patient's reasonable goals, values, and priorities and falls within the boundaries of medical standards of care, institutional policy, and legal mandates and prohibitions.
      - [ ] **Decision**: The patient's or surrogate's decision has been communicated to the appropriate individuals, documented in the medical records, and shared with all relevant healthcare team members.

2. **Practitioner Beneficence** (Maximize Benefits):
    - **Specification**: Practitioner has determined that beneficence is being implemented with the treatment options that will be presented to the patient.
    - **Beneficence's Necessary Conditions:**
      (all boxes must be checked for compliance)
      - ☐ **Maximization**: The practitioner's treatment options maximize the patient's best interests, as determined by the patient's reasonable goals, values, and priorities.
      - ☐ **Boundaries**: The practitioner's treatment options comply with medical standards of care, institutional policies, and legal mandates and prohibitions.
      - ☐ **Review**: Decisions to maximize benefits should be revisited regularly as patient conditions and circumstances change.

---

3. **Practitioner Nonmaleficence** (Minimize Burdens):
    - **Specification**: Practitioner has determined that nonmaleficence is being implemented with the treatment options that will be presented to the patient.
    - **Nonmaleficence's Necessary Conditions:**
      (all boxes must be checked for compliance)
      - ☐ **Minimization**: The practitioner's treatment options minimize the patient's burdens, as determined by the patient's reasonable goals, values, and priorities.
      - ☐ **Boundaries**: The practitioner's treatment options comply with medical standards of care, institutional policies, and legal mandates and prohibitions.

4. **Public Justice** (Ensure Fairness):
   - **Specification**: Practitioner determines that justice as fairness is being implemented.
   - **Justice's Necessary Conditions:**
     (all boxes must be checked for compliance)
     - ☐ **Fairness**: The practitioner's treatment options promote fairness.
     - ☐ **Boundaries**: The practitioner's treatment options comply with medical standards of care, institutional policies, and legal mandates and prohibitions.

---

## (C) CONCLUDE

- ☐ **Weigh**: The patient/surrogate and practitioner must jointly determine the relative weights of each of the four specified principles, considering the patient's reasonable goals, values, and priorities, medical standards of care, institutional policies, and legal mandates and prohibitions.
- ☐ **Balance**: The patient/surrogate and practitioner must jointly determine which principle, or groups of principles, guide the decision-making towards a rational and reasonable recommendation or decision.
- ☐ **Communicate**: Clearly document and communicate the agreed-upon decision to all relevant parties to ensure understanding and alignment.

**DOCUMENTATION:**

**SOAP Notes:**

- ☐ **(S) Subjective**: Document the patient's or surrogate's perspective on the medical condition, diagnosis, prognosis, and treatment options, including their ethical considerations.
- ☐ **(O) Objective**: Record objective medical facts, such as diagnosis, clinical observations, and test results. Ensure all facts align with current medical standards of care.
- ☐ **(A) Assessment**: Evaluate the ethical issues identified, summarizing the THINK and ASSESS steps, and document the TAC analysis with reference to each bioethical principle.
- ☐ **(P) Plan**: Develop a plan that outlines the recommended course of action, including steps for communicating findings and recommendations to all stakeholders. Document how the decision adheres to ethical principles, medical standards of care, and legal requirements.

**Consultant Name:** ______________________________
**Date:** ___________

## 4.3 SOAP Notes

---

**Purpose:** To provide a comprehensive and structured format for documenting ethics consultations using the SOAP (Subjective, Objective, Assessment, Plan) method.

**Consultation Date:** [Date]
**Consultant:** [Name/Title]
**Patient/Case ID:** [ID]
**Department:** [Department Name]

---

### — (S) Subjective

#### Patient's Perspective

- **Narrative**: Document the patient's understanding of their medical condition, goals, values, and concerns.

  **Open-ended Questions:**

  - "Can you tell me about your understanding of your current medical condition?"
  - "What are your goals and priorities regarding your treatment?"
  - "How do you feel about the proposed medical interventions?"
  - "Are there any specific concerns or values that are particularly important to you in making healthcare decisions?"

#### Family's Perspective

- **Narrative**: Document the family's understanding, goals, and concerns regarding the patient's condition and treatment.

  **Open-ended Questions:**

  - "Can you share your thoughts and concerns about your loved one's medical condition and treatment?"
  - "What are your goals and priorities for your loved one's care?"

- "How do you think your loved one feels about their current situation and the proposed treatments?"
- "How do you think your loved one's values and priorities should guide the decisions being made?"

**PRACTITIONERS' PERSPECTIVE**

- **Narrative**: Document the practitioners' views on the medical condition, treatment plan, and ethical considerations.

  **Open-ended Questions:**

  - "Can you explain the medical condition and proposed treatment plan?"
  - "What do you see as the primary benefits and risks of the proposed interventions?"
  - "How do you incorporate the patient's values and preferences into the treatment plan?"
  - "Is the proposed treatment plan in alignment with current healthcare standards of care, institutional policies, and professional guidelines?"
  - "How do you ensure that the treatment plan reflects the patient's reasonable goals, values, and priorities?"

---

## — (O) Objective

**Medical Facts:**

- **Summary**: Provide an overview of the patient's medical condition, diagnosis, and prognosis.
- **Clinical Data**: Include relevant medical history, current treatments, and proposed interventions.
- **Observations**: Note any observations related to the patient's condition and interactions with staff.
- **Alignment**: Ensure that all medical facts align with current medical healthcare standards of care.

## — (A) Assessment

**Ethical Issues Identified:**

- **Patient Autonomy** (informed consent)**:**
  - Assess the patient's capacity to make informed decisions.
  - Document the information provided to the patient about treatment options.
- **Practitioner Beneficence** (promote benefits)**:**
  - Evaluate the potential benefits of the proposed interventions.
- **Practitioner Nonmaleficence** (avoid harm)**:**
  - Identify potential risks and harms associated with the treatments.
- **Public Justice** (promote fairness)**:**
  - Consider fairness in the allocation of resources and treatment options.
- **Alignment with Medical Standards of Care:**
  - Ensure proposed treatment plans adhere to current medical healthcare standards.
- **Patient's Reasonable Goals, Values, and Priorities:**
  - Ensure these are central to the ethical analysis and treatment plan.
- **Compliance with Professional, Institutional, State, and Federal Standards:**
  - Verify that the treatment plan complies with relevant laws, policies, and social expectations.

---

## — (P) Plan

**Ethical Recommendations**:

- **Steps**: Outline specific steps to address the identified ethical issues.
- **Communication**: Include a plan for further communication with the patient, family, and practitioners.

- **Decisions**: Document any decisions made during the consultation.

**Follow-up:**

- **Meetings**: Schedule follow-up meetings to reassess the situation and ensure implementation of ethical recommendations.
- **Responsibilities**: Assign responsibilities to team members for monitoring the patient's condition and ethical aspects of care.

**Documentation:**

- **EHR**: Ensure all discussions, decisions, and plans are thoroughly documented in the patient's Electronic Health Record (EHR).
- **Alignment**: Confirm that documentation reflects alignment with current healthcare standards, the patient's reasonable goals, values, and priorities, and compliance with professional, institutional, state, and federal standards.

**Signature:** [Consultant's Signature]
**Date:** [Date]

***

## 4.4 SOAP Notes—Cue Card

### (S) Subjective

Patient:
- Understand condition?
- Goals and priorities?
- Feelings about treatment?
- Important values/concerns?

Family:
- Thoughts/concerns?
- Goals for loved one?
- Loved one's values/priorities?

Practitioners:
- Condition/treatment explanation?
- Benefits/risks?
- Alignment with standards of care?
- Patient's values/preferences?

### (O) Objective

- Medical condition/prognosis
- Treatments/interventions
- Standards of care/compliance

### (A) Assessment

Ethical analysis:
- Ethical issues (Autonomy, Beneficence, Nonmaleficence, Justice)
- Alignment with medical standards of care
- Patient's Reasonable Goals, Values, and Priorities
- Compliance with Professional, Institutional, State, and Federal mandates

### (P) Plan

Action steps:
- Address issues
- Communicate plan
- Document decisions
- Follow-up schedule
- Compliance with medical standards of care

***

## 4.5 Post-Consultation Survey

**Purpose**: To collect standardized and quantifiable data on the effectiveness of the ethics consultation process from participants.

**Survey Design:**

**Question Types:**

- **Likert Scale Questions**: Provides a quantitative measure of satisfaction with various aspects of the consultation process..
- **Multiple Choice Questions**: Collects specific information on the outcomes and procedural aspects of the consultation.
- **Open-Ended Questions**: Gathers qualitative feedback that provides deeper insights into participants' experiences and perspectives.

**Distribution:**

- **Timing**: Send the survey within 24-48 hours after the consultation to ensure that experiences are fresh in participants' minds.
- **Delivery Method**: Use online survey tools (e.g., SurveyMonkey, Google Forms) for easy distribution and data collection. For those less comfortable with digital tools, consider paper surveys as an alternative.

**Response Tracking:**

- **Anonymity Option**: Offer participants the option to submit responses anonymously to encourage honest feedback
- **Response Rate Monitoring**: Track response rates and send reminders to non-respondents to ensure a representative sample of feedback.

Here are several examples for each question type in a post-consultation survey designed to gather structured feedback on the ethics consultation process. They will provide a well-rounded approach to collecting structured feedback, which can be used to improve the ethics consultation proccss continuously.

## I. Likert Scale Questions

**Purpose**: Measure participants' satisfaction with different aspects of the consultation process.

**Satisfaction with Timeliness:**

A. How satisfied were you with the timeliness of the ethics consultation?

1. Very Dissatisfied
2. Dissatisfied
3. Neutral
4. Satisfied
5. Very Satisfied

**Clarity of Communication:**

B. How clear was the communication from the ethics consultant during the consultation?

1. Very Unclear
2. Unclear
3. Neutral
4. Clear
5. Very Clear

**Effectiveness of Resolution:**

C. How effective was the ethics consultation in resolving the ethical issue at hand?

1. Very Ineffective
2. Ineffective
3. Neutral
4. Effective
5. Very Effective

**Respect for Participants' Perspectives:**

D. To what extent did the ethics consultant respect and consider your perspective during the consultation?

1. Not at All
2. Slightly
3. Neutral

4. Considerably
5. Completely

**Overall Satisfaction:**

E. Overall, how satisfied were you with the ethics consultation process?

1. Very Dissatisfied
2. Dissatisfied
3. Neutral
4. Satisfied
5. Very Satisfied

## II. Multiple Choice Questions

**Purpose:** Gather specific information on outcomes or decisions made during the consultation.

**Resolution of Ethical Dilemma:**

1. Did the ethics consultation help resolve the ethical issue to your satisfaction?
   a) Yes
   b) Partially
   c) No

**Understanding of Ethical Principles:**

2. After the consultation, how well do you feel you understand the ethical principles involved?
   a) Very Well
   b) Somewhat Well
   c) Not Very Well
   d) Not at All

**Consultation Duration:**

3. Was the duration of the ethics consultation appropriate for addressing the issue?
   a) Yes, it was appropriate
   b) No, it was too short
   c) No, it was too long

**Follow-up Actions:**

4. Were clear follow-up actions or recommendations provided at the end of the consultation?
   a) Yes, clear actions were provided
   b) Yes, but the actions were somewhat unclear
   c) No, no clear actions were provided

**Involvement in Decision-Making:**

5. Do you feel that you were adequately involved in the decision-making process during the consultation?
   a) Yes, fully involved
   b) Somewhat involved
   c) Not involved at all

## III. Open-Ended Questions

**Purpose**: Allow participants to provide detailed feedback on their experience.

**Suggestions for Improvement:**

- What suggestions do you have for improving the ethics consultation process?

**Unresolved Issues:**

- Were there any aspects of the ethical issue that you feel were not adequately addressed? If so, please explain.

**Experience with the Ethics Consultant:**

- Can you describe your experience with the ethics consultant? Were there any specific qualities or actions that you found particularly helpful or unhelpful?

**Impact on Care:**

- How did the ethics consultation impact the care or treatment plan? Please provide details.

**General Feedback:**

- Is there anything else you would like to share about your experience with the ethics consultation process?

***

## 4.6 Follow-Up Interview

**Purpose**: To explore the nuances of participants' experiences and gather qualitative data that may not be captured through surveys. This guide is designed for semi-structured interviews, allowing for flexibility in responses while ensuring key topics are covered.

## Interview Guide for Follow-Up Interviews on Ethics Consultations

This guide allows for flexibility in the interview process while ensuring that all critical areas are explored. The open-ended nature of the questions encourages participants to share their experiences in detail, providing valuable qualitative data that can be used to enhance the ethics consultation process.

### I. Introduction

- **Opening Statement:**
  "Thank you for taking the time to participate in this interview. The purpose of this conversation is to gain a deeper understanding of your experience with the recent ethics consultation. Your insights will help us improve the process and ensure that it meets the needs of all involved. This interview is confidential, and your responses will be anonymized in any reporting. Do you have any questions before we begin?"
- **Consent Confirmation:**
  "Do I have your permission to record this interview for accuracy in transcribing your responses?"

### II. Background Information

- **Participant Role:**
  "Could you please describe your role in the ethics consultation? Were you the patient, a family member, a healthcare provider, or an ethics consultant?"

- **Context of the Consultation:**
"Can you briefly describe the ethical issue that was addressed during the consultation?"

**III. Key Topics and Questions**

**1. Impact on Decision-Making**

*Question*: "Can you describe how the ethics consultation impacted your decision-making process? Did it change or reinforce your initial thoughts?"

*Follow-Up*: "Were there any specific recommendations or insights from the consultation that particularly influenced your decision?"

**2. Satisfaction with the Process**

*Question*: "How satisfied were you with the overall consultation process?"

*Follow-Up*: "Was there anything about the process that you found particularly helpful or unhelpful?"

**3. Clarity and Communication**

*Question*: "How clear was the communication from the ethics consultant during the consultation? Did you feel that the ethical issues were explained in an understandable way?"

*Follow-Up*: "Were there any aspects that were confusing or difficult to understand?"

**4. Respect and Consideration**

*Question*: "Do you feel that your perspective and concerns were respected and taken into account during the consultation?"

*Follow-Up*: "Was there anything more that could have been done to ensure that your views were considered?"

**5. Outcomes and Resolutions**

*Question*: "Were you satisfied with the outcomes or resolutions that resulted from the ethics consultation?"

*Follow-Up*: "Did the consultation provide a clear path forward, or were there any unresolved issues?"

**6. Challenges Encountered**

*Question*: "Did you encounter any challenges during the consultation process? If so, could you describe them?"
*Follow-Up*: "How do you think these challenges could be addressed in future consultations?"

**7. Suggestions for Improvement**
*Question*: "Do you have any suggestions for how the ethics consultation process could be improved?"
*Follow-Up*: "Is there anything specific that you think should be added, removed, or changed?"

## IV. Open-Ended Closing Questions

- **General Experience:**
"Is there anything else you would like to share about your experience with the ethics consultation that we haven't covered?"

- **Final Thoughts:**
"Do you have any final thoughts or reflections on the consultation process that you believe are important for us to consider?"

## V. Conclusion

- **Closing Statement:**
"Thank you very much for sharing your insights. Your feedback is invaluable in helping us improve our ethics consultation process. If you have any further thoughts after this interview, please feel free to reach out to us."

- **Next Steps:**
"We will be compiling feedback from these interviews to identify areas for improvement. If you are interested in learning about the outcomes of our review, we can provide a summary of the findings once the process is complete."

- **Confirm Contact Information** (if necessary)**:**
"Could you please confirm your preferred contact information in case we need to follow up with any clarifications?"

**Interview Notes**

- **Transcription**: Record and transcribe the interview, noting any significant points or recurring themes.
- **Analysis**: Use the transcribed data to identify key insights, patterns, and areas for improvement that can inform changes to the ethics consultation process.

***

## 4.7 Feedback Forms

**Purpose**: To allow participants to express their thoughts and concerns freely, without fear of repercussions, especially in sensitive cases.

**Form Design**

- **Simple and Direct**: Keep the feedback form short and to the point, with prompts that encourage candid responses (e.g., "Please share any concerns or suggestions you have regarding the ethics consultation.").
- **Anonymity Assurance**: Clearly state that the feedback form is anonymous, and no identifying information will be collected.

**Distribution**

- **Placement**: Make feedback forms available in multiple locations (e.g., at the end of the consultation, in follow-up emails, or on the program's website).
- **Accessibility**: Ensure that forms are easy to fill out and submit, with both physical drop boxes and online submission options.

**Analysis**

- **Regular Review**: Collect and review feedback forms regularly to identify patterns and areas needing attention.
- **Actionable Insights**: Focus on feedback that offers actionable insights, and incorporate this into continuous improvement efforts.

## Anonymous Feedback Form for Ethics Consultation

This anonymous feedback form is designed to be simple and direct, encouraging candid responses while assuring participants of their anonymity. By keeping the questions straightforward and offering open text fields for additional comments, the form aims to gather honest and constructive feedback that can be used to enhance the ethics consultation process.

**Purpose**: This form is designed to allow you to provide anonymous feedback on your experience with the ethics consultation process. Your responses are confidential, and no identifying information will be collected. Your honest feedback is crucial in helping us improve the quality and effectiveness of our ethics consultations.

**Feedback Form**

**1. Overall Experience**

"How would you rate your overall experience with the ethics consultation process?"

- ☐ Excellent
- ☐ Good
- ☐ Fair
- ☐ Poor

**2. Clarity of Communication**

"Did you find the communication during the ethics consultation clear and easy to understand?"

- ☐ Yes, very clear
- ☐ Somewhat clear
- ☐ Not clear

**3. Respect for Your Perspective**

"Did you feel that your perspective and concerns were respected during the consultation?"

- ☐ Yes
- ☐ No
- ☐ Unsure

**4. Resolution of Ethical Issue**

"Was the ethical issue addressed to your satisfaction?"

- ☐ Yes, fully addressed
- ☐ Partially addressed
- ☐ Not addressed

**5. Suggestions for Improvement**

"Please share any concerns or suggestions you have regarding the ethics consultation process."
[Open Text Field]

**6. Additional Comments**

"Is there anything else you would like to add about your experience with the ethics consultation?"
[Open Text Field]

**Anonymity Assurance**

Please note: This feedback form is completely anonymous. We do not collect any personal or identifying information. Your responses will be used solely for the purpose of improving our ethics consultation process. Thank you for your candid feedback.

**Instructions for Submission**

- **Online Submission**: If completing this form online, please click "Submit" when finished.
- **Paper Submission**: If completing a paper form, please place it in the designated drop box located [insert location], or return it to the specified office.

**Thank You**

"Thank you for taking the time to provide your feedback. Your insights are invaluable in helping us ensure that our ethics consultations are conducted with the highest standards of care and respect."

***

## Further Readings and References

**Overview of Healthcare Ethics Consultations**

- Aulisio, M. P., Arnold, R. M., & Youngner, S. J. (2003). Health Care Ethics Consultation: Theory, Practice, and Cases. Johns Hopkins University Press.
  - *Provides a comprehensive overview of healthcare ethics consultations, combining theoretical insights with practical case studies to illustrate best practices in the field.*
- Dubler, N. N., & Liebman, C. B. (2011). Bioethics Mediation: A Guide to Shaping Shared Solutions. United Hospital Fund of New York.
  - *Focuses on the mediation aspect of bioethics, offering guidance on how to facilitate shared solutions in ethical disputes within healthcare settings.*

**Strategies for Effective Consultations**

- La Puma, J., & Schiedermayer, D. L. (1994). Ethics Consultation: A Practical Guide. Jones and Bartlett Publishers.
  - *A practical guide offering step-by-step strategies for conducting effective ethics consultations, including communication techniques and decision-making frameworks.*
- Slowther, A., Johnston, C., Goodall, J., & Hope, T. (2004). Development of clinical ethics committees. BMJ, 328(7445), 950-952.
  - *Discusses the establishment and development of clinical ethics committees, highlighting their role in supporting effective ethics consultations.*

**Case Studies and Real-world Examples**

- Jonsen, A. R., & Toulmin, S. E. (1988). The Abuse of Casuistry: A History of Moral Reasoning. University of California Press.
  - *Examines the historical and philosophical development of casuistry and its application in clinical ethics, providing valuable case studies and examples.*

- Rhodes, R., & Alfandre, D. (2007). A systematic approach to clinical moral reasoning. Clinical Ethics, 2(2), 66-70.
    - *Introduces a systematic approach to clinical moral reasoning, illustrated with real-world case studies to enhance understanding of practical ethical decision-making.*

***

# Chapter 5: Policy Development and Organizational Ethics

## Developing and Reviewing Policies

Policy development is fundamental to the Bioethics Program, serving as a cornerstone for addressing ethical issues, ensuring consistency in decision-making, and promoting ethical awareness across the healthcare organization. The director's role in leading policy development and review is crucial, involving collaboration with legal, clinical, and administrative teams to create policies that are ethically robust, legally compliant, and practically applicable. Policies should reflect the core bioethical principles of patient autonomy (informed consent), practitioner beneficence (maximize benefits), practitioner nonmaleficence (minimize burdens), and public justice (ensure fairness). These principles must be balanced with institutional policies, established medical standards of care, and legal mandates.

### Key Principles in Policy Development:

1. **Patient Autonomy** (Informed Consent):
   Policies must ensure that patients, or their legally established surrogates when patients lack decisional capacity, are provided with all the necessary information to make informed decisions. This includes understanding the diagnosis and prognosis, knowing all available treatment options (including no treatment), comprehending the purpose of each option, and evaluating the benefits and risks. Surrogates must use substituted judgment when making medical decisions on behalf of the patient. Patients or surrogates should also be able to articulate logical reasons for their choices, ensuring these align with the patient's reasonable goals, values, and priorities and patients or surrogates must clearly communicate voluntary consent or rejection of treatment options.

2. **Practitioner Beneficence** (maximize benefits):
   Policies should guide healthcare practitioners to maximize the benefits to patients by recommending treatment options that align with the patient's reasonable goals, values, and priorities. This alignment ensures the provision of care that enhances the patient's well-being, taking into account their unique circumstances and preferences. Practitioners must be supported in understanding and applying these principles while adhering to medical standards of care, institutional policies, and legal requirements.
3. **Practitioner Nonmaleficence** (Minimize Burdens):
   Policies must emphasize the importance of avoiding unnecessary harm to patients. This involves careful evaluation of potential risks associated with any treatment options and ensuring that harm is minimized. Practitioners should be guided to make decisions that respect patient autonomy while prioritizing the avoidance of harm, in alignment with ethical standards and legal mandates.
4. **Public Justice** (Ensure Fairness):
   Policies should incorporate the principle of justice, ensuring that healthcare decisions are fair and equitable. This includes considering the broader implications of healthcare decisions on society, the fair allocation of resources, and ensuring that all patients receive equitable treatment regardless of their background or circumstances. Policies must align with legal frameworks and institutional standards to uphold the principle of fairness in all aspects of patient care and organizational practice.

## Steps for Policy Development

Identify Ethical Issues: Start by identifying key ethical issues that the policy aims to address. This involves consulting relevant ethical guidelines, medical standards, and legal requirements.

- **Collaborate with Stakeholders**: Engage with stakeholders, including legal experts, clinicians, ethics consultants, and patient representatives, to gather diverse perspectives and insights. This collaborative approach ensures that the policy is comprehensive, practical, and reflective of the needs and values of all involved parties.

- **Draft Clear and Comprehensive Policies**: Policies should be written in plain language, avoiding technical jargon to ensure they are accessible to all practitioners. They must provide practical guidance for addressing ethical issues, specifying procedures for obtaining informed consent, evaluating treatment options, and documenting decision-making processes.
- **Regular Review and Revision**: Establish a schedule for regular review and revision of policies to maintain their relevance and effectiveness. This process should involve gathering feedback from practitioners, reviewing recent ethics consultations, and staying informed about changes in regulations and best practices. Regular updates ensure that policies continue to support ethical decision-making and compliance.
- **Continuous Feedback Mechanisms**: Create channels for practitioners to provide feedback on policies, such as suggestion boxes, surveys, or regular meetings. Continuous feedback helps identify practical challenges or unintended consequences of policies, allowing for timely adjustments and improvements.

### Ensuring Compliance with Regulatory Standards and Ethical Norms:

- **Legal and Ethical Alignment:** Policies must align with relevant laws, regulations, and professional guidelines. The director should stay informed about changes in healthcare regulations and ethical standards, engaging with legal and compliance experts to ensure that all policies are current and compliant.

- **Fostering Ethical Awareness**: Promoting a culture of ethical awareness and responsibility is essential. This includes providing regular training and education on ethical issues, facilitating discussions and reflections on ethical dilemmas, and recognizing ethical behavior. A culture of ethics enhances the overall ethical climate of the organization.
- **Monitoring and Enforcement**: Implement mechanisms for monitoring adherence to policies, such as regular audits and accountability systems. Monitoring ensures that policies are consistently applied, and any breaches are promptly identified and addressed. Enforcement actions should be clearly defined and communicated to maintain accountability.
- **Integration with Quality Improvement**: Compliance efforts should be integrated with the organization's broader quality improvement initiatives. Aligning compliance activities with patient safety programs and risk management helps create a holistic approach to quality and ethics.

### Case Study: Informed Consent Policy Development

- **Purpose and Scope**: The development of an informed consent policy is crucial for ensuring that patients make well-informed decisions about their care. This policy should provide clear guidelines for obtaining and documenting consent, especially in complex cases involving vulnerable populations or high-risk procedures.
- **Stakeholder Engagement**: Engage with legal experts, clinicians, ethics consultants, and patient representatives to gather input and ensure that the policy reflects diverse perspectives. Collaborative development helps build support and ensures the policy addresses practical challenges faced by practitioners.
- **Implementation and Communication**: Ensure that the informed consent policy is effectively implemented and communicated. This includes providing training to

practitioners, creating templates and checklists for documenting consent, and establishing mechanisms for monitoring and evaluating compliance.

- **Ongoing Evaluation**: Establish mechanisms for continuous evaluation and improvement of the informed consent policy. Regular feedback from practitioners and patients, along with audits of consent documentation, will help identify areas for improvement and ensure the policy remains effective and relevant.
- **Promoting a Culture of Informed Consent**: Foster an environment where patients are encouraged to ask questions and participate actively in their care decisions. By promoting a culture of informed consent, the organization can enhance patient autonomy, trust, and overall satisfaction with care.

**Conclusion**:

Aligning policy development with the mission and vision of the Bioethics Program is critical for promoting ethical decision-making, patient autonomy, and compliance with legal and institutional standards. By emphasizing the four core bioethical principles and ensuring that policies are clear, accessible, and regularly reviewed, the Bioethics Program can enhance the quality and compassion of patient care. This alignment fosters an ethical culture that supports the best interests of patients and the integrity of the healthcare organization.

***

The following forms and templates provide a comprehensive toolkit to support the development, review, implementation, and monitoring of policies within the Bioethics Program. They are designed to ensure that policies are clear, practical, and aligned with both legal requirements and ethical standards, ultimately enhancing the effectiveness of the Bioethics Program.

***

## 5.1/15.1 Policy Development Template

**Purpose**: To provide a structured and comprehensive framework for developing, implementing, and maintaining clear, legally compliant, and ethically robust policies within the organization.

**Policy Title:** [Title of the Policy]
**Policy Number:** [Assign a unique policy number]
**Date of Creation/Revision:** [Date the policy was created or last revised]
**Effective Date:**[Date the policy comes into effect]
**Review Date:** [Scheduled date for the policy review]

**Purpose**

- Clearly state the purpose of the policy, including its objectives, the issues it addresses, and what it aims to achieve within the organization.

**Scope**

- Define the scope of the policy, including:
  - The individuals, departments, or processes to which the policy applies.
  - Any specific circumstances or contexts under which the policy is applicable.

**Definitions**

- Provide clear definitions for any key terms used within the policy to ensure understanding and consistency in interpretation.

**Policy Statement**

- Articulate the core principles, ethical standards, and key guidelines upon which the policy is based. This section should be a concise declaration of the policy's intentions and overarching framework.

**Procedures**

- Detail the specific steps required to implement and comply with the policy. This should include:
  - **Step-by-Step Guidelines:** A detailed description of the procedures to be followed.
  - **Documentation Requirements:** Outline any forms, checklists, or documentation that must be completed as part of the process.

**Responsibilities**

- Clearly assign and describe the roles and responsibilities of individuals or departments involved in the implementation and oversight of the policy.

**Legal, Ethical, and Compliance Considerations**

- Identify and discuss any relevant laws, regulations, ethical guidelines, or institutional standards that the policy must adhere to. Ensure that the policy aligns with both legal and ethical requirements.

**Training and Education**

- Describe any training or educational initiatives required to effectively implement the policy. Specify the target audience, training content, and delivery methods.

**Monitoring, Compliance, and Evaluation**

- Outline the mechanisms for monitoring adherence to the policy, including:
  - **Compliance Monitoring:** Methods for ensuring that the policy is followed, such as audits or reporting requirements.
  - **Evaluation:** Processes for assessing the effectiveness of the policy and its impact.
  - **Enforcement:** Describe any enforcement actions or consequences for non-compliance.

**Review and Revision Process**

- Detail the process for reviewing and revising the policy, including:

- **Frequency of Review:** How often the policy should be reviewed.
- **Process for Revision:** Steps for making revisions, including who is responsible for the review and how revisions will be approved.

**Related Policies and Documents**

- List any related policies, procedures, or documents that should be consulted in conjunction with this policy to ensure comprehensive coverage of the subject matter.

**Approval**

- Include a section for formal approval, noting the authorities responsible for finalizing and approving the policy.

**Approved by:** [Name and Title]
**Date of Approval:** [Approval Date]

**Appendices**

- Attach or reference any supplementary documents, forms, or additional materials that support the policy.

***

## 5.2 Policy Development, Review, and Revision Checklist

**Purpose:** To ensure that policies are effectively developed, regularly reviewed, updated, and remain relevant to the organization's goals, compliance requirements, and operational needs.

**Policy Title:** [Title of the Policy]
**Policy Number:** [Policy Number]
**Date:** [Date of Creation/Revision]
**Review Conducted By:** [Name/Title of the Reviewer]
**Next Review Date:** [Scheduled Date of Next Review]

1. **Purpose**
   - ☐ Are the policy's objectives clearly stated and aligned with the organization's goals?
   - ☐ Does the policy still address a current and relevant issue?
2. **Scope**
   - ☐ Is the target audience for the policy clearly defined?
   - ☐ Does the policy comprehensively cover all affected parties and situations?
3. **Definitions**
   - ☐ Are all key terms clearly defined?
   - ☐ Is there consistency with existing policies and terminology?
4. **Procedures**
   - ☐ Are the procedures detailed, clear, and practical for implementation?
   - ☐ Do the procedures remain applicable and effective?
5. **Responsibilities**
   - ☐ Are specific roles and responsibilities clearly assigned?
   - ☐ Is accountability for actions and decisions well established?

6. **Compliance and Enforcement**
   - ☐ Does the policy comply with current laws, regulations, and ethical guidelines?
   - ☐ Are the monitoring and enforcement mechanisms still effective?
   - ☐ Are there any consequences for non-compliance outlined clearly?
7. **Effectiveness**
   - ☐ Has the policy been effective in achieving its intended outcomes?
   - ☐ Are there any gaps, weaknesses, or unintended consequences that need addressing?
8. **Stakeholder Feedback**
   - ☐ Has feedback from stakeholders (e.g., practitioners, patients, legal experts) been considered?
   - ☐ Have practical challenges identified by stakeholders been addressed?
9. **Training and Implementation**
   - ☐ Is additional training or resources required to support the policy's implementation?
   - ☐ Are there any barriers to effective implementation that need to be addressed?
10. **References**
    - ☐ Are relevant laws, guidelines, and external standards included?
    - ☐ Is the policy consistent with external references and internal standards?
11. **Appendices**
    - ☐ Are all supplementary materials, forms, and templates attached?

12. **Final Review and Approval**
    - ☐ Has the policy been reviewed by all necessary stakeholders?
    - ☐ Is the policy ready for approval by the relevant authorities?
    - ☐ Are there any additional comments or recommendations for changes to the policy?
13. **Action Taken**
    - ☐ Describe any actions taken as a result of the review, including revisions, updates, or the decision to maintain the current policy.

***

## 5.3 Policy Implementation and Communication

**Purpose**: To outline the steps required to effectively communicate and implement a new or revised policy within the organization.

**Policy Title**: [Title of the Policy]
**Policy Number**: [Policy Number]
**Effective Date**: [Date the policy comes into effect]
**Implementation Lead**: [Name/Title of the person responsible for implementation]

**Communication Strategy**:

- Identify the key audiences who need to be informed about the policy.
- Outline the methods for communicating the policy (e.g., email, staff meetings, intranet, training sessions).
- Specify any key messages or talking points to be included in the communication.

**Training and Resources**:

- Describe any training sessions or materials needed to ensure that staff understand and can apply the policy.
- Identify who will be responsible for delivering the training and by when it should be completed.

**Implementation Timeline**:

- Providc a timeline for the key activities required to implement the policy, including communication, training, and any necessary preparations.

**Monitoring and Support**:

- Outline the methods for monitoring the implementation of the policy, including follow-up surveys, compliance checks, or additional support sessions.

- Identify the resources or support available to staff during the implementation process.

**Feedback and Adjustment**:

- Describe how feedback will be gathered from staff during the implementation process and how it will be used to make any necessary adjustments to the policy or its application.

**Reporting**:

- Identify who will be responsible for reporting on the implementation progress to senior management and when these reports will be made.

***

## 5.4 Informed Consent Policy Template

**Purpose**: To provide a clear and comprehensive template for developing a policy on informed consent, ensuring that all legal, ethical, and practical considerations are addressed.

**Policy Title**: Informed Consent Policy
**Policy Number**: [Assign a unique policy number]
**Effective Date**: [Date the policy comes into effect]
**Review Date**: [Scheduled date for policy review]

**Purpose**:

To ensure that informed consent is obtained and documented for all medical procedures and treatments, in compliance with legal and ethical standards.

**Scope**:

- This policy applies to all healthcare practitioners and practitioners involved in obtaining consent from patients within [Institution's Name].

**Definitions**:

- *Informed Consent*: The process by which a patient with decisional capacity is informed about the available treatment opitions, including no treatment, and the risks, benefits, associated with each alternative and the patient makes a voluntary decision.

**Policy Statement**:

- All patients must be provided with clear, comprehensive information about their treatment options and must voluntarily consent before any procedure is performed.

**Procedures**:

- Obtaining Consent:
  - Provide information in a manner that is understandable to the patient.
  - Ensure that consent is given voluntarily, without coercion.
  - Document the consent process thoroughly in the patient's medical record.
- Special Considerations:
  - Additional steps for vulnerable populations (e.g., minors, cognitively impaired patients).
  - Procedures for obtaining consent in emergency situations.
- Documentation:
  - Use standardized forms for documenting informed consent.
  - Ensure that all relevant details, including discussions of risks and alternatives, are recorded.

- Legal and Ethical Considerations:
- Ensure compliance with applicable laws and regulations regarding informed consent.
- Incorporate ethical principles of autonomy, beneficence, and nonmaleficence in the consent process.

**Training and Implementation**:

- Provide training for all practitioners on the informed consent process, including legal and ethical requirements.
- Create resources and tools (e.g., checklists, templates) to support practitioners in obtaining and documenting consent.

**Monitoring and Compliance**:

- Conduct regular audits of consent documentation to ensure compliance.
- Provide feedback and additional training as needed.

**Review and Revision Process**:

- Schedule regular reviews of the informed consent policy, with input from legal, clinical, and patient representatives.
- Update the policy as needed to reflect changes in laws, ethical standards, or organizational practices.

**Approval**:

- Approval by [Names/Titles of Approving Authorities].

***

## 5.5 Policy Feedback Form

**Purpose**: To gather continuous feedback from practitioners on the effectiveness and practicality of existing policies.

**Policy Title**: [Title of the Policy]
**Policy Number**: [Policy Number]
**Date**: [Date of Feedback Submission]
**Role**: [Practitioner's Role/Department]

**Understanding of the Policy**

1. How clear is the policy in terms of its language and instructions?
   - ☐ Very Clear
   - ☐ Somewhat Clear
   - ☐ Not Clear
   - ☐ Confusing

**Practicality of the Policy**

2. How practical is the policy in your daily work?
   - ☐ Very Practical
   - ☐ Somewhat Practical
   - ☐ Not Practical
   - ☐ Impractical

**Challenges Encountered**

3. Have you encountered any challenges in implementing this policy?
   - ☐ Yes
   - ☐ No

   If Yes, please describe the challenges:
   [Open Text Field]

**Suggestions for Improvement**

4. Do you have any suggestions for improving this policy?
   [Open Text Field]

**Additional Comments**

5. Is there anything else you would like to share regarding this policy?
   [Open Text Field]

**Submission**:

- Please submit this form to [Designated Person/Department] or place it in the designated policy feedback box.

***

## Further Readings and References

### Developing and Reviewing Policies

- American College of Healthcare Executives. (2011). Policy Development Handbook. ACHE.
    - *A comprehensive handbook on developing and reviewing healthcare policies, providing essential guidance for bioethics program directors.*
- Moreno, J. D. (2005). Is There an Ethicist in the House? On the Cutting Edge of Bioethics. Indiana University Press.
    - *Explores contemporary issues in bioethics and the role of ethicists in policy development and organizational ethics, offering insights into effective policy-making.*

### Ensuring Compliance with Regulatory Standards and Ethical Norms

- Annas, G. J. (2011). Worst Case Bioethics: Death, Disaster, and Public Health. Oxford University Press.
    - *Analyzes the intersection of bioethics, public health, and regulatory standards, emphasizing the importance of compliance in organizational ethics.*
- Childress, J. F. (2007). Public Bioethics: Principles and Problems. Oxford University Press.
    - *Examines the principles and challenges of public bioethics, offering guidance on ensuring ethical and regulatory compliance in healthcare organizations.*

### Informed Consent Policy Development

- Faden, R. R., Beauchamp, T. L., & King, N. M. P. (1986). A History and Theory of Informed Consent. Oxford University Press.
    - *Provides a historical and theoretical overview of informed consent, illustrating the development and implementation of informed consent policies.*

- Miller, F. G., & Wertheimer, A. (2010). The Ethics of Consent: Theory and Practice. Oxford University Press.
  - *Explores the ethical dimensions of consent, offering practical guidance on the development of informed consent policies in healthcare.*


***

# Chapter 6: Preventive Ethics

## Importance of Preventive Ethics

Preventive ethics is a proactive approach aimed at identifying and addressing ethical issues before they escalate into significant problems. This approach is vital for fostering ethical awareness, promoting ethical decision-making, and preventing ethical breaches and conflicts. The Bioethics Program's mission and vision statements emphasize the integration of core bioethical principles—patient autonomy (informed consent), practitioner beneficence (maximize benefits), practitioner nonmaleficence (minimize burdens), and public justice (ensure fairness)—in all aspects of healthcare delivery. Preventive ethics aligns with these principles by ensuring that ethical considerations are proactively managed, enhancing the overall ethical climate and improving patient care.

## Core Principles in Preventive Ethics:

1. **Patient Autonomy** (Informed Consent):
   Preventive ethics ensures that patient autonomy is respected and upheld by facilitating informed consent processes. This includes ensuring that patients or their legally established surrogates understand their medical condition, know all available treatment options (including the option of no treatment), comprehend the purpose of each treatment, and can evaluate the benefits and risks of these options. By proactively addressing potential ethical dilemmas around consent, such as communication barriers or decisional capacity, preventive ethics helps safeguard the patient's right to make informed choices aligned with their reasonable goals, values, and priorities.

2. **Practitioner Beneficence** (maximize benefits):
   Practitioners are committed to promoting the well-being of patients. Preventive ethics encourages healthcare providers to

consider the potential benefits of various interventions early in the decision-making process. By focusing on maximizing patient benefits, preventive ethics aligns with the commitment to enhancing the patient's well-being according to their reasonable goals and values, within the context of medical standards of care and institutional policies.

3. **Practitioner Nonmaleficence** (Minimize Burdens):
A key tenet of preventive ethics is the avoidance of harm. This involves identifying potential risks and ethical issues before they arise, thereby minimizing harm to patients. Preventive ethics strategies, such as ethics rounds and early warning systems, help identify and mitigate risks, ensuring that healthcare decisions do not cause unnecessary harm. This proactive approach aligns with the principle of nonmaleficence and the commitment to providing care that does not compromise patient safety.

4. **Public Justice** (Ensure Fairness):
Preventive ethics supports fairness in healthcare by addressing systemic issues that may lead to ethical dilemmas. By ensuring that policies and practices are equitable and just, preventive ethics promotes public justice. This involves recognizing and mitigating disparities in care, ensuring that all patients receive fair and equal treatment, and considering the broader implications of healthcare decisions on society. Preventive ethics thus supports the ethical climate of the organization and promotes a culture of fairness.

## Implementing Preventive Ethics Strategies:

- **Ethics Rounds**:
Regular ethics rounds are a cornerstone of preventive ethics. These sessions allow healthcare teams to discuss real or hypothetical cases, identify potential ethical issues, and explore solutions before problems escalate. Ethics rounds should be interdisciplinary, involving clinicians, administrators, ethics consultants, and other stakeholders. By fostering open dialogue and ethical reflection, these sessions

help practitioners develop their ethical reasoning skills and ensure that ethical considerations are integrated into clinical practice.

- **Training and Education**:
  Continuous education on ethical principles and decision-making is essential for preventive ethics. Training sessions should be interactive and cover a wide range of topics, including informed consent, end-of-life care, confidentiality, and cultural competence. These sessions should equip practitioners with the skills and knowledge to recognize and respond to ethical issues proactively. The Bioethics Program should provide regular opportunities for training, ensuring that all healthcare providers are aware of their ethical responsibilities and the tools available to support ethical practice.

- **Early Warning Systems**:
  Developing and implementing early warning systems is a key component of preventive ethics. These systems help identify ethical issues before they become critical. Tools such as ethical risk assessments, incident reporting systems, and ethics audits can be used to monitor for potential ethical concerns. Early intervention allows for timely resolution, preventing ethical breaches and conflicts. The director should ensure that these systems are user-friendly, accessible, and effectively integrated into the organization's broader quality improvement initiatives.

## Fostering a Culture of Ethical Vigilance:

- **Promoting Ethical Awareness**:
  The director should promote a culture of ethical vigilance, where practitioners are continuously aware of and attuned to ethical issues. This involves creating an environment that encourages ethical reflection, dialogue, and the continuous identification of ethical challenges. Regularly scheduled ethics

rounds, accessible training programs, and opportunities for ethical discussion should be standard practice.

- **Encouraging Reporting and Feedback**:
  A culture of openness where practitioners feel safe to report ethical concerns is crucial. This can be achieved through confidential reporting mechanisms and regular feedback channels, such as suggestion boxes or anonymous surveys. Practitioners should be encouraged to speak up about potential ethical issues without fear of retribution. Feedback from these channels can inform policy development and help refine preventive ethics strategies.

- **Celebrating Ethical Behavior**:
  Recognizing and celebrating ethical behavior reinforces the importance of ethics in healthcare. This can involve acknowledging practitioners who demonstrate ethical excellence or creativity in resolving ethical dilemmas. Such recognition not only promotes a positive ethical culture but also encourages others to prioritize ethical considerations in their practice.

## Addressing Systemic Issues

- **Identifying Trends**:
  The director should regularly review data from ethics consultations, incident reports, and feedback to identify trends and recurring issues. Understanding these patterns helps to address systemic issues that may lead to ethical dilemmas. By implementing preventive measures to tackle these root causes, the organization can reduce the occurrence of ethical conflicts.

- **Developing Policies and Procedures**:
  Policies and procedures should be developed to address identified ethical issues and prevent their recurrence. These policies must be in line with the organization's mission and vision, emphasizing the core bioethical principles and compliance with legal and institutional standards. Regular

review and revision of these policies ensure they remain effective and relevant.

- **Integration with Organizational Ethics**:
  Preventive ethics should be integrated into the broader organizational ethics framework, ensuring alignment with quality improvement and risk management programs. This holistic approach to ethics supports the overall mission of the Bioethics Program, promoting ethical decision-making at all levels of the organization.

## Monitoring and Evaluation

- **Continuous Evaluation**:
  The effectiveness of preventive ethics activities should be regularly evaluated. This involves gathering feedback from practitioners, reviewing ethics consultations, and conducting audits. Continuous evaluation helps identify areas for improvement and ensures that preventive ethics activities are aligned with the Bioethics Program's mission and vision.
- **Feedback Mechanisms**:
  Practitioners should be encouraged to provide feedback on the preventive ethics strategies. Regular feedback ensures that the strategies remain relevant and effective, and allows for the timely adjustment of policies and procedures. Feedback can be collected through surveys, focus groups, and individual consultations.
- **Policy Review**:
  The director should establish a schedule for the regular review of preventive ethics policies. Involving a diverse group of stakeholders in this process ensures that policies are comprehensive and reflect the evolving ethical landscape of healthcare. Regular review helps maintain the relevance and effectiveness of policies, supporting the Bioethics Program's goals.

## Conclusion

Preventive ethics plays a critical role in aligning healthcare practices with the core bioethical principles of patient autonomy (informed consent), practitioner beneficence (maximize benefits), practitioner nonmaleficence (minimize burdens), and public justice (ensure fairness). By implementing proactive strategies such as ethics rounds, training sessions, and early warning systems, the Bioethics Program can promote ethical awareness, prevent ethical conflicts, and enhance patient care. The integration of preventive ethics into the broader organizational framework supports a culture of ethical vigilance and responsibility, ensuring that ethical considerations are central to all aspects of healthcare delivery.

***

The following forms and templates provide practical tools to support the implementation and monitoring of preventive ethics strategies. By utilizing these resources, the Bioethics Program can proactively address ethical issues, promote ethical awareness, and foster a culture of ethical vigilance within the organization. These tools will help in identifying and addressing ethical issues before they escalate, promoting a proactive approach to ethics within the organization.

***

## 6.1 Ethics Rounds Discussion Template

**Purpose**: To facilitate structured and productive ethics rounds, allowing participants to explore ethical issues in a systematic way.

**Date**: [Date of Ethics Rounds]
**Facilitator**: [Name of the Facilitator]
**Participants**: [List of Participants and their Roles]

**Case Description:**

- Briefly describe the case being discussed, including relevant medical, ethical, and contextual details.

**Key Ethical Issues**:

- Identify and list the primary ethical issues involved in the case (e.g., informed consent, patient autonomy, end-of-life decisions).

**Discussion Points**:

- What are the different perspectives on the ethical issues?
- What ethical principles are in conflict?
- How might these conflicts be resolved?

**Decision-Making Process**:

- What decision-making framework or model is being used to address the ethical issues?
- How are the ethical principles being weighed and balanced in this case?

**Recommendations**:

- What are the recommended actions or resolutions for the case?
- How should these recommendations be communicated and implemented?

**Follow-Up Actions**:

- List any follow-up actions that need to be taken, including additional consultations, policy reviews, or training needs.

**Reflections**:

- Encourage participants to reflect on what they learned from the discussion and how it might apply to their practice.

**Next Steps**:

- Schedule the next ethics rounds session and identify any topics or cases for future discussion.

***

## 6.2 Ethical Risk Assessment Form

**Purpose**: To identify potential ethical risks in clinical practice or organizational policies before they become critical issues.

**Date**: [Date of Assessment]
**Assessor**: [Name/Title of the Assessor]
**Department/Unit**: [Department or Unit Being Assessed]

**Area of Focus:**

- Specify the area of focus for the risk assessment (e.g., informed consent processes, end-of-life care, confidentiality practices).

**Identified Risks:**

- List any potential ethical risks identified during the assessment.

**Risk Level:**

- Assess the level of risk associated with each identified issue (e.g., low, medium, high).

**Contributing Factors:**

- Identify any factors contributing to the risk (e.g., lack of training, unclear policies, resource constraints).

**Recommended Preventive Measures:**

- Provide recommendations for addressing or mitigating the identified risks.

**Implementation Plan:**

- Outline the steps required to implement the recommended preventive measures, including timelines and responsible parties.

**Monitoring and Follow-Up:**

- Describe how the effectiveness of the preventive measures will be monitored and when follow-up assessments will occur.

**Comments:**

- Include any additional observations or considerations relevant to the assessment.

***

## 6.3 Incident Reporting Form for Ethical Concerns

**Purpose**: To provide a mechanism for practitioners to report ethical concerns or incidents as part of an early warning system.

**Date of Incident**: [Date]
**Reported By**: [Name/Title - Optional for anonymity]
**Department/Unit**: [Department or Unit Involved]

**Description of Incident:**

- Provide a detailed description of the incident or ethical concern, including relevant context and individuals involved.

**Ethical Issues Involved:**

- Identify the specific ethical issues raised by the incident (e.g., conflict of interest, breach of confidentiality, informed consent).

**Immediate Actions Taken:**

- Describe any immediate actions taken to address the ethical concern.

**Suggestions for Resolution:**

- Provide any suggestions or recommendations for resolving the issue.

**Follow-Up Needed:**

- Indicate whether further investigation or follow-up is required and what steps should be taken.

**Confidentiality:**

- State any concerns about confidentiality and how they should be handled.

**Submitted To**: [Name/Title of the Person or Committee to whom the report is submitted]

***

## 6.4 Preventive Ethics Activity Log

**Purpose**: To document and monitor ongoing preventive ethics activities, ensuring that they are tracked and evaluated over time.

**Activity Name**: [Name of the Preventive Ethics Activity]
**Date**: [Date of Activity]
**Coordinator**: [Name/Title of the Activity Coordinator]

**Description:**

- Briefly describe the preventive ethics activity (e.g., ethics rounds, training session, ethics audit).

**Objectives:**

- List the primary objectives of the activity (e.g., raising ethical awareness, identifying potential ethical issues, promoting ethical decision-making).

**Participants:**

- List the participants involved in the activity.

**Outcomes:**

- Describe the outcomes of the activity, including any issues identified, lessons learned, or recommendations made.

**Follow-Up Actions:**

- List any follow-up actions required as a result of the activity.

**Feedback:**

- Document any feedback received from participants or stakeholders about the activity.

**Next Steps:**

- Outline the next steps for this preventive ethics activity or related initiatives.

**Review Date**: [Date for Reviewing the Effectiveness of the Activity]

***

## 6.5 Ethics Audit Checklist

**Purpose**: To systematically review and evaluate ethics practices within the organization as part of a preventive ethics strategy.

**Audit Date**: [Date]
**Auditor(s)**: [Name(s) and Title(s) of the Auditor(s)]
**Department/Unit**: [Department or Unit Being Audited]

**Checklist Items:**

1. **Ethics Consultation Processes**:
   - Are ethics consultations documented thoroughly?
   - Are ethical principles consistently applied in decision-making?
   - Are there any recurring ethical issues that need to be addressed?
2. **Informed Consent Procedures**:
   - Are informed consent processes being followed correctly?
   - Are patients provided with clear and understandable information?
   - Is consent documented properly?
3. **Confidentiality Practices**:
   - Are patient confidentiality and privacy maintained consistently?
   - Are there any breaches of confidentiality that need to be addressed?
4. **Conflict of Interest Management**:
   - Are potential conflicts of interest identified and managed appropriately?
   - Are there clear policies in place for addressing conflicts of interest?

5. **Ethical Training and Education**:
   - Are staff regularly trained on ethical principles and practices?
   - Is there evidence of ongoing ethical education and awareness activities?
6. **Reporting and Accountability**:
   - Are there clear mechanisms for reporting ethical concerns?
   - Is there a system in place for holding individuals accountable for ethical breaches?

**Audit Findings:**

- Document the findings of the audit, including any areas of concern or good practice.

**Recommendations:**

- Provide recommendations for improving ethics practices based on the audit findings.

**Action Plan:**

- Develop an action plan for implementing the recommendations, including timelines and responsible parties.

**Follow-Up Audit Date**: [Date for the Follow-Up Audit]

***

## Further Readings and References

### Importance of Preventive Ethics


- Foglia, M. B., Pearlman, R. A., Bottrell, M., Altemose, J., & Fox, E. (2009). Preventive ethics: Addressing ethics quality gaps on a systems level. The Joint Commission Journal on Quality and Patient Safety, 35(7), 318-324.
  - *Discusses the concept of preventive ethics and its application at the systems level to address and prevent ethical issues in healthcare.*
- Roberts, L. W. (2009). The Ethical Dimension of Psychological Practice. American Psychological Association.
  - *Explores the ethical considerations in psychological practice, emphasizing the importance of preventive ethics in maintaining high standards of ethical conduct.*


### Strategies for Proactive Ethics Activities


- DuVal, G., Sartorius, L., Clarridge, B., Gensler, G., & Danis, M. (2001). What triggers requests for ethics consultations? Journal of Medical Ethics, 27(suppl 1), i24-i29.
  - *Investigates the common triggers for ethics consultations, providing insights into proactive strategies to address potential ethical dilemmas before they escalate.*
- Tarzian, A. J., & The ASBH Core Competencies Update Task Force. (2013). Health care ethics consultation: An update on core competencies and emerging standards from the American Society for Bioethics and Humanities' Task Force on Standards for Bioethics Consultation. The American Journal of Bioethics, 13(2), 3-13.
  - *Updates on core competencies and emerging standards in healthcare ethics consultation, offering guidance on proactive ethics activities to prevent ethical issues.*

**Implementing Early Warning Systems for Ethical Dilemmas**

- Fox, E., Myers, S., & Pearlman, R. A. (2007). Ethics consultation in United States hospitals: A national survey. The American Journal of Bioethics, 7(2), 13-25.
  - *Presents the findings of a national survey on ethics consultation in U.S. hospitals, highlighting the importance of early warning systems for identifying and addressing ethical dilemmas.*
- Wolf, S. M. (2010). The role of ethics committees in public health. Journal of Law, Medicine & Ethics, 38(3), 718-726.
  - *Examines the role of ethics committees in public health, emphasizing their function in implementing early warning systems and preventing ethical issues.*

***

# Review Questions

**True/False Questions:**

1. Healthcare ethics consultations often address complex issues such as end-of-life decisions, conflicts between patients and providers, and questions of informed consent.
True or False?

2. The role of the Bioethics Program Director includes establishing clear protocols for initiating and conducting ethics consultations.
True or False?

3. It is unnecessary for the Bioethics Program Director to stay informed about current ethical standards and best practices.
True or False?

4. Effective ethics consultations require a interprofessional approach, involving input from various stakeholders.
True or False?

5. Regular evaluation and feedback loops are not necessary for maintaining the integrity of the ethics consultation process.
True or False?

**Multiple-Choice Questions:**

6. What is an essential element in the process of conducting healthcare ethics consultations?
a) Ignoring the perspectives of patients and families
b) Gathering and considering all relevant information
c) Avoiding the documentation of consultation outcomes
d) Restricting input to only medical professionals

7. Which of the following is NOT a key responsibility of a Bioethics Program Director during ethics consultations?
a) Providing leadership and oversight for the Bioethics Program
b) Facilitating open and respectful discussions
c) Ignoring systemic issues that give rise to ethical dilemmas
d) Educating and training practitioners on ethical principles

**Clinical Vignettes:** '

8. A patient is unable to make informed decisions due to cognitive impairment, and the family disagrees with the healthcare team's proposed treatment plan. What is the best course of action for the Bioethics Program Director?
a) Ignore the family's concerns
b) Facilitate a meeting to discuss the perspectives and find a resolution
c) Side with the healthcare team without discussion
d) Recommend the family seek legal action

9. A nurse raises an ethical concern about a physician's decision to withhold critical information from a patient about their prognosis. What should the Bioethics Program Director do?
a) Tell the nurse to follow the physician's orders
b) Review the situation and discuss the ethical implications with the healthcare team
c) Ignore the concern
d) Advise the nurse to find another job

10. During a healthcare ethics consultation, it becomes evident that a hospital policy is contributing to recurring ethical conflicts. What is the best approach for the Bioethics Program Director?
a) Ignore the issue and continue with the current policy
b) Analyze the policy and work to implement preventive measures to address the underlying causes
c) Advise practitioners to avoid discussing the policy
d) Remove the policy without any review

## Correct Answers:

1. True
2. True
3. False (It is necessary for the Bioethics Program Director to stay informed about current ethical standards and best practices.)
4. True
5. False (Regular evaluation and feedback loops are necessary for maintaining the integrity of the ethics consultation process.)
6. b) Gathering and considering all relevant information
7. c) Ignoring systemic issues that give rise to ethical dilemmas
8. b) Facilitate a meeting to discuss the perspectives and find a resolution
9. b) Review the situation and discuss the ethical implications with the healthcare team
10. b) Analyze the policy and work to implement preventive measures to address the underlying causes

***

# Part III: Enhancing Communication and Education

## Chapter 7: Effective Communication in Ethics Consultation

Effective communication is foundational to ethics consultations and integral to the Bioethics Program's mission and vision. By focusing on the core bioethical principles—patient autonomy (informed consent), practitioner beneficence (maximize benefits), practitioner nonmaleficence (minimize burdens), and public justice (ensure fairness)—effective communication helps ensure that ethical considerations are central to patient care and decision-making. This chapter expands on techniques for active listening and empathetic engagement, the mediation of conflicts, and providing clear and balanced ethical advice, ensuring these align with established medical standards, institutional policies, and legal mandates.

### Techniques for Active Listening and Empathetic Engagement

**Active Listening**:

Active listening is the bedrock of effective communication in ethics consultations. It involves fully engaging with the speaker, understanding their concerns, and responding in a way that confirms their message has been heard. Active listening requires practitioners to:

1. **Give Full Attention**: Practitioners should focus entirely on the speaker, minimizing distractions. This helps in building trust and ensures that the speaker feels respected and valued.

2. **Ask Clarifying Questions**: Practitioners should ask questions that help clarify the speaker's statements, ensuring a clear understanding of their concerns and perspectives. For example, "Could you explain what concerns you most about this treatment option?"
3. **Reflect Back**: Practitioners should summarize and reflect back what has been said to confirm understanding. Phrases such as, "What I'm hearing is…" or "It sounds like you're saying…" can be used to ensure accuracy and understanding.

### Empathetic Engagement

Empathy is crucial for understanding and validating the emotions and experiences of others. It involves:

1. **Recognizing Emotions**: Practitioners should acknowledge the emotions expressed by patients, families, or colleagues. Statements like, "I can see that this is very difficult for you," validate the speaker's feelings and demonstrate empathy.
2. **Responding with Compassion**: Empathetic engagement requires practitioners to respond in a way that shows care and concern for the speaker's emotional state. Compassionate responses can help de-escalate emotional situations and foster a supportive environment.
3. **Supporting and Empowering**: Empathetic engagement also means empowering patients and families to express their values and concerns openly, contributing to informed decision-making processes that align with their reasonable goals and priorities.

### Training and Development

The Bioethics Program should include comprehensive training in active listening and empathetic engagement as part of professional development. This can involve:

1. **Practical Exercises and Role-Playing**: Simulated patient interviews and role-playing scenarios provide practitioners with

opportunities to practice these skills in a controlled, supportive environment.

2. **Feedback and Reflection**: Providing structured feedback sessions after role-playing exercises allows practitioners to reflect on their performance and identify areas for improvement. Reflection helps practitioners internalize these skills and understand their impact on patient care.
3. **Workshops and Refresher Courses**: Regular workshops and refresher courses help maintain these skills, ensuring they remain sharp and relevant. These sessions should be mandatory for new hires and scheduled regularly for existing practitioners.
4. **Ongoing Practice and Support**: Creating opportunities for regular practice through team meetings, peer support groups, and mentorship programs encourages continuous improvement. Practitioners can discuss their communication challenges and successes, learning from each other's experiences.

## Mediating Conflicts and Facilitating Consensus

Conflicts often arise in ethics consultations due to differing goals, values, and priorities among stakeholders. These conflicts might involve disagreements between patients and healthcare providers, between family members, or within the healthcare team itself. Effective mediation helps resolve these conflicts and aligns decision-making with the bioethical principles.

## Key Mediation Techniques

1. **Creating a Safe Environment:** The director should ensure that all parties feel safe and respected during discussions. Establishing ground rules for respectful communication can prevent escalations and facilitate constructive dialogue.
2. **Helping Articulate Concerns**: Practitioners should help each party articulate their concerns and viewpoints. This involves using active listening to fully understand each perspective and encouraging open communication.

3. **Exploring Solutions**: Practitioners should guide discussions towards exploring potential solutions that align with the patient's reasonable goals, values, and priorities while adhering to medical standards, institutional policies, and legal requirements.
4. **Facilitating Consensus**: Practitioners should aim to find common ground and facilitate a resolution that all parties can accept. This requires balancing firmness and flexibility, maintaining neutrality, and being prepared to offer ethical advice based on the core bioethical principles.

## Training in Mediation Skills

To enhance the ability to mediate conflicts, the Bioethics Program should provide targeted training that includes:

1. **Role-Playing Scenarios**: Practical exercises where practitioners take on different roles in simulated conflict situations help them develop mediation skills in a realistic context.
2. **Feedback and Guidance**: Providing feedback on mediation techniques and strategies helps practitioners refine their skills and become more effective mediators.
3. **Ongoing Practice and Reflection**: Regular debriefings after ethics consultations allow practitioners to reflect on their mediation experiences, discuss challenges, and share effective strategies.
4. **Developing Mediation Protocols**: The director should establish clear protocols for mediation during ethics consultations. These protocols should outline steps for conflict resolution, define the roles and responsibilities of each participant, and provide criteria for evaluating the success of the mediation.

## Ensuring Clear and Balanced Ethical Advice

Ethics consultations must provide clear and balanced ethical advice that considers all perspectives and aligns with the core bioethical principles. Effective ethical advice involves:

1. **Thorough Ethical Analysis:** Practitioners must conduct a comprehensive analysis of each case, considering the ethical dimensions and applying relevant principles, such as patient autonomy, beneficence, nonmaleficence, and justice.
2. **Clarity and Accessibility**: Ethical advice should be communicated clearly and concisely, avoiding jargon or overly technical language. The use of plain language ensures that all stakeholders understand the advice provided.
3. **Balancing Risks and Benefits**: Ethical advice should offer a balanced view, considering both the benefits and risks of different options. Practitioners should explain the rationale behind their recommendations, helping stakeholders make informed decisions.
4. **Supporting Ethical Decision-Making**: Ethical advice should empower stakeholders to make decisions that align with the patient's reasonable goals, values, and priorities, while ensuring compliance with medical standards, institutional policies, and legal mandates.

### Documentation and Protocols

To ensure consistency and quality in ethical advice, the Bioethics Program should implement:

1. **Templates and Checklists**: Standardized templates for documenting ethics consultations can ensure thorough analysis and clear communication. These templates should include sections for outlining ethical principles, summarizing stakeholder perspectives, and detailing the recommended course of action.
2. **Training on Documentation**: Practitioners should be trained in documenting ethics consultations effectively, ensuring transparency and accountability.
3. **Regular Audits and Feedback**: The director should establish a system for regularly reviewing consultation records and

providing feedback to practitioners. This helps maintain high standards and identifies areas for improvement.

4. **Staying Informed:** The director and practitioners should stay updated on developments in bioethics and healthcare law to ensure that advice remains current and relevant. This can involve attending conferences, participating in professional organizations, and keeping up with literature in the field.

## Promoting a Culture of Ethical Awareness

To enhance the effectiveness of ethical advice and consultations, the Bioethics Program should foster a culture of ethical awareness through:

1. **Continuous Learning and Improvement**: Regular training and education on ethical principles and decision-making help practitioners stay informed and improve their skills.
2. **Opportunities for Discussion and Reflection**: Regular team meetings, ethics rounds, and debriefing sessions provide opportunities for practitioners to discuss ethical dilemmas and learn from each other's experiences.
3. **Recognition of Ethical Excellence**: Acknowledging practitioners who demonstrate ethical excellence reinforces the importance of ethics in healthcare and encourages others to prioritize ethical considerations in their practice.

## Conclusion

Enhancing communication and education in ethics consultations is essential for aligning with the Bioethics Program's mission and vision. By developing skills in active listening, empathetic engagement, conflict mediation, and providing clear ethical advice, the program ensures that ethical considerations are central to patient care and decision-making. Continuous training, reflection, and adherence to bioethical principles, institutional policies, and legal mandates will support the ongoing effectiveness and integrity of the Bioethics Program.

***

The following forms and templates provide essential tools for enhancing communication skills, mediating conflicts, and ensuring clear and balanced ethical advice during ethics consultations. By utilizing these resources, the Bioethics Program can improve the effectiveness of its consultations and promote a culture of open, empathetic, and ethical communication within the organization.

***

## 7.1 Active Listening and Empathetic Engagement Training Worksheet

**Purpose**: To guide practitioners through exercises that enhance active listening and empathetic engagement skills.

**Date**: [Date of Training]
**Participant Name**: [Name of Participant]
**Facilitator**: [Name of Facilitator]

**Exercise 1: Active Listening Practice**

**Scenario**:

- Describe a hypothetical or real scenario where active listening is critical (e.g., a patient expressing concerns about a treatment plan).

**Listening Techniques**:

- Focus on the speaker without interrupting.
- Use non-verbal cues (e.g., nodding, eye contact) to show attentiveness.
- Paraphrase or reflect back what the speaker has said to ensure understanding.

**Reflection**:

- How did using active listening techniques change your understanding of the speaker's concerns?
- What challenges did you encounter while practicing active listening?

**Exercise 2: Empathetic Engagement Role-Play**

**Scenario**:

- Describe a scenario where empathetic engagement is needed (e.g., a family member expressing grief or frustration).

**Empathy Techniques**:

- Acknowledge and validate the emotions expressed.
- Use compassionate language and tone.
- Offer support without judgment or assumptions.

**Reflection**:

- How did practicing empathetic engagement impact the interaction?
- What strategies helped you connect with the other person emotionally?

**Feedback from Facilitator:**

- Provide personalized feedback on the participant's performance in both exercises, highlighting strengths and areas for improvement.

***

## 7.2 Mediation and Conflict Resolution Protocol

**Purpose**: To provide a structured approach for mediating conflicts and facilitating consensus during ethics consultations.

**Date**: [Date of Consultation]
**Facilitator**: [Name of Mediator]
**Participants**: [List of Participants]

**Conflict Summary:**

- Briefly describe the conflict, including the key issues and stakeholders involved.

**Step 1: Creating a Safe Environment**

- Ensure all participants feel respected and heard.
- Establish ground rules for the discussion (e.g., no interruptions, respectful language).

**Step 2: Articulation of Concerns**

- Allow each participant to articulate their concerns without interruption.
- Use active listening to ensure each perspective is fully understood.

**Step 3: Identifying Common Goals**

- Identify any shared goals or values among the participants (e.g., patient well-being, upholding ethical standards).

**Step 4: Exploring Solutions**

- Facilitate a discussion on potential solutions, encouraging creativity and compromise.
- Ensure that all options are explored and evaluated against ethical principles.

**Step 5: Reaching Consensus**

- Guide the group toward a mutually acceptable resolution.
- Summarize the agreed-upon solution and ensure all participants understand the next steps.

**Follow-Up Actions:**

- List any actions required to implement the resolution, including responsible parties and timelines.

**Evaluation of Mediation Success:**

- Assess the effectiveness of the mediation process. Did the resolution meet the ethical standards and address the concerns of all parties?

**Reflections and Lessons Learned:**

- Encourage participants to reflect on what they learned from the mediation process and how it might apply to future cases.

***

## 7.3 Ethics Consultation Summary Template

**Purpose**: To document and communicate the key points and outcomes of an ethics consultation in a clear and balanced manner.

**Date of Consultation**: [Date]
**Consultant(s)**: [Name(s) of Ethics Consultant(s)]

**Case Overview:**

- Provide a brief summary of the case, including relevant clinical and ethical details.

**Key Ethical Issues:**

- Identify the primary ethical issues involved in the case (e.g., autonomy, beneficence, confidentiality).

**Stakeholder Perspectives:**

- Summarize the perspectives of the key stakeholders (e.g., patient, family, healthcare team).

**Ethical Analysis:**

- Apply relevant ethical principles and guidelines to the case. Discuss the benefits and risks of different options.

**Recommendations:**

- Provide clear and balanced recommendations, explaining the rationale behind each suggestion.

**Conclusion:**

- Summarize the consultation's conclusions, including any agreements reached and next steps.

**Follow-Up Actions:**

- List any follow-up actions required, including timelines and responsible parties.

**Reviewer's Notes:**

- Include any additional comments or reflections from the ethics consultant or reviewing authority.

***

## 7.4 Reflective Practice and Peer Feedback Form

**Purpose**: To facilitate reflection and peer feedback on communication skills following an ethics consultation.

**Date**: [Date of Reflection]
**Participant Name**: [Name of Participant]
**Peer Reviewer**: [Name of Peer Reviewer]

**Reflection on Communication:**

**Active Listening:**

- Reflect on how well you practiced active listening during the consultation.
- What challenges did you face, and how did you address them?

**Empathetic Engagement:**

- Reflect on your ability to engage empathetically with the stakeholders.
- How did this affect the consultation process and outcomes?

**Mediation and Conflict Resolution:**

- Reflect on any conflicts that arose during the consultation. How effectively were they mediated?
- What strategies did you use to facilitate consensus?

**Peer Feedback:**

**Strengths:**

- What communication strengths did you observe in your peer during the consultation?

**Areas for Improvement:**

- What aspects of their communication could be improved? Provide constructive suggestions.

**Overall Assessment:**

- Overall, how effective was your peer in facilitating the consultation?

**Action Plan:**

- Based on your reflection and peer feedback, identify one or two areas for improvement and outline a plan to address them.

***

## 7.5 Communication Skills Workshop Evaluation Form

**Purpose**: To evaluate the effectiveness of communication skills workshops and gather feedback for future improvement.

**Workshop Title**: [Title of the Workshop]
**Date**: [Date of Workshop]
**Facilitator**: [Name of Facilitator]

1. **Workshop Content:**
   How relevant and useful was the content presented in the workshop?
   ☐ Very Relevant
   ☐ Somewhat Relevant
   ☐ Not Relevant
2. **Practical Exercises:**
   How effective were the practical exercises (e.g., role-playing, simulations) in enhancing your communication skills?
   ☐ Very Effective
   ☐ Somewhat Effective
   ☐ Not Effective
3. **Facilitator's Effectiveness:**
   How effective was the facilitator in delivering the workshop content and guiding discussions?
   ☐ Very Effective
   ☐ Somewhat Effective
   ☐ Not Effective
4. **Key Takeaways:**
   - What were the most important takeaways from the workshop?
5. **Suggestions for Improvement:**
   - Do you have any suggestions for improving this workshop or future communication skills training sessions?

**6. Additional Comments:**

- Is there anything else you would like to share about your experience with this workshop?

***

## Further Readings and References


### Techniques for Active Listening and Empathetic Engagement

- Brown, J. B. (2008). The Use of Active Listening and Empathy in Clinical Encounters. Oxford University Press.
  - *Explores the crucial skills of active listening and empathy in clinical settings, providing practical techniques for improving patient communication and understanding.*
- Hunsaker, R. A. (2010). The Art of Empathy: A Training Course in Life's Most Essential Skill. Sounds True.
  - *Offers a comprehensive training course on developing empathy, highlighting its importance and application in both personal and professional interactions.*

### Mediating Conflicts and Facilitating Consensus

- Fisher, R., Ury, W. L., & Patton, B. (2011). Getting to Yes: Negotiating Agreement Without Giving In (3rd ed.). Penguin Books.
  - *Presents principles and strategies for effective negotiation and conflict resolution, emphasizing win-win solutions and collaborative approaches.*
- Moore, C. W. (2014). The Mediation Process: Practical Strategies for Resolving Conflict (4th ed.). Jossey-Bass.
  - *Provides a detailed guide to the mediation process, offering practical strategies and techniques for resolving conflicts and facilitating consensus in diverse settings.*

### Ensuring Clear and Balanced Ethical Advice

- Pellegrino, E. D., & Thomasma, D. C. (1993). The Virtues in Medical Practice. Oxford University Press.
  - *Examines the role of virtues in medical practice and their significance in providing clear and ethically sound advice in clinical ethics consultations.*

- Thompson, I. E. (1996). Philosophical Approaches to Medical Ethics. University of Toronto Press.
  - *Explores various philosophical approaches to medical ethics, providing a solid theoretical foundation for offering balanced and well-reasoned ethical advice.*


***

# Chapter 8: Designing and Delivering Ethics Education Programs

Ethics education is a cornerstone of the Bioethics Program, ensuring that healthcare practitioners are equipped with the knowledge, skills, and ethical framework necessary to make informed and ethically sound decisions. This chapter outlines strategies for designing and delivering engaging and effective ethics education programs, emphasizing the integration of the four core bioethical principles—patient autonomy (informed consent), practitioner beneficence (maximize benefits), practitioner nonmaleficence (minimize burdens), and public justice (ensure fairness). The chapter also discusses the importance of aligning educational content with institutional policies, established medical standards of care, and legal mandates to support the Bioethics Program's mission and vision.

## Creating Engaging and Effective Training Sessions

To ensure ethics education is both engaging and effective, training sessions should incorporate a variety of interactive teaching methods tailored to the specific needs of the audience. The following strategies should be employed:

1. **Lectures and Discussions**: While lectures provide a foundation of knowledge, incorporating discussions encourages participants to engage actively with the material. Facilitators should pose open-ended questions and encourage dialogue, allowing participants to explore ethical concepts and their applications.

2. **Case Studies**: Real-world case studies are invaluable for illustrating the complexities of ethical dilemmas. These should reflect diverse clinical scenarios and challenge participants to apply ethical principles. Case studies should include elements of patient autonomy, beneficence, nonmaleficence, and justice,

allowing participants to practice balancing these principles in decision-making.

3. **Simulations and Role-Playing**: Simulations provide a safe environment for participants to practice their ethical decision-making skills. Role-playing scenarios, especially those involving surrogate decision-making, can help participants understand different perspectives and the application of substituted judgment. These activities should be designed to reflect realistic situations that practitioners may encounter, ensuring relevance to clinical practice.
4. **Interactive Technology**: Utilizing technology such as virtual reality (VR), augmented reality (AR), and interactive online platforms can enhance engagement. These tools can simulate complex ethical scenarios, offering immersive experiences that deepen understanding and retention.

### Tailoring Content to the Audience

Ethics education should be relevant and applicable to the daily responsibilities of the participants. The director should consider the following:

1. **Audience-Specific Content**: Training should be customized based on whether participants are clinical practitioners, administrators, students, or other stakeholders. For example, sessions for clinicians might focus on patient consent and end-of-life care, while training for administrators could cover policy development and ethical oversight.
2. **Cultural Competence**: Addressing cultural, religious, and social factors is critical in ethics education. Training should include discussions on how these factors influence patient values and ethical decision-making. This helps practitioners provide culturally sensitive care that respects patient autonomy.
3. **Ethical Principles Integration**: Each training session should integrate the four core bioethical principles. Scenarios should be selected to highlight the importance of informed consent, the

balance of benefits and harms, and the need for fairness in healthcare decisions.

## Ongoing Learning and Development

To foster continuous improvement and lifelong learning, the director should provide opportunities for ongoing ethics education:

1. **Online Training Modules**: Developing online resources, including webinars, e-learning courses, and digital libraries, allows for flexible learning. These resources should be accessible to all staff and updated regularly to reflect the latest ethical guidelines and best practices.
2. **Resource Availability**: Providing access to relevant articles, books, and case studies encourages self-directed learning. A well-curated library of resources can support practitioners in staying informed about emerging ethical issues.
3. **Reflection and Debriefing**: Incorporating reflective practices into training sessions, such as journaling or group discussions, helps participants process their experiences and understand the ethical implications of their actions. Regular debriefing sessions after ethics consultations can serve as ongoing learning opportunities.

## Using Interactive Workshops, Case Studies, and Simulations

Interactive tools are essential for effective ethics education. They allow participants to engage actively with ethical concepts and practice applying them in realistic scenarios.

1. **Workshops**: Interactive workshops provide a collaborative space for discussing ethical issues. These should be structured to encourage active participation, with a focus on real-life ethical dilemmas. Participants can share experiences, discuss challenges, and develop their ethical reasoning skills.
2. **Case Studies**: Carefully selected case studies should illustrate the application of bioethical principles in various contexts. The

director should choose cases that highlight common ethical challenges, such as informed consent issues, conflicts of interest, and allocation of scarce resources. Each case should be accompanied by guided questions to stimulate critical thinking and discussion.

3. **Simulations**: Simulations offer hands-on experience in handling ethical issues. By recreating real-world scenarios, simulations allow participants to practice decision-making, communication, and conflict resolution skills. Feedback from facilitators and peers during simulations helps reinforce learning and identify areas for improvement.

## Incorporating Technology in Interactive Education

The use of technology can enhance the effectiveness of workshops, case studies, and simulations:

1. **Virtual Reality (VR) and Augmented Reality (AR)**: VR and AR can create immersive environments where participants experience ethical scenarios firsthand. These technologies can simulate patient interactions, complex decision-making processes, and the perspectives of different stakeholders, enhancing empathy and understanding.
2. **Online Platforms**: Interactive online platforms enable real-time collaboration and discussion, making them ideal for conducting virtual workshops and case studies. These platforms can include features such as breakout rooms, polling, and interactive whiteboards to facilitate engagement.

## Evaluating and Improving Education Programs

Regular evaluation is crucial for maintaining the quality and relevance of ethics education programs. The director should implement a comprehensive evaluation strategy:

1. **Participant Feedback**: Gathering feedback through surveys, interviews, and informal discussions helps assess the effectiveness of training sessions. Feedback should focus on

content relevance, engagement levels, and the applicability of learned skills to real-world situations.

2. **Quantitative and Qualitative Methods**: Combining quantitative methods (e.g., pre- and post-training assessments) with qualitative feedback provides a holistic view of the program's impact. This approach helps identify knowledge gaps and areas needing improvement.
3. **Regular Reviews**: The director should review training materials, records, and feedback regularly. This ensures that content remains current and reflects best practices and emerging trends in bioethics.

## Incorporating Best Practices and Emerging Trends

To keep ethics education programs dynamic and responsive, the director should:

1. **Stay Informed**: Attend professional conferences, participate in training programs, and engage with professional organizations to stay updated on the latest developments in ethics education. Networking with peers can provide new ideas and perspectives.
2. **Adapt and Innovate**: Incorporate new teaching methods, technologies, and content based on feedback and emerging trends. Being adaptable ensures that the Bioethics Program remains relevant and effective in an ever-evolving healthcare environment.

## Conducting Research to Measure Impact

Formal research can provide valuable insights into the effectiveness of ethics education programs. The director should consider:

1. **Collaborating with Academic Institutions**: Partnering with universities or research organizations can facilitate studies on the impact of ethics education. Research can focus on measuring changes in participants' knowledge, attitudes, and behaviors following training.

2. **Publishing Findings**: Sharing research findings through publications and presentations can contribute to the broader field of ethics education and highlight the Bioethics Program's commitment to excellence.

**Conclusion**

Designing and delivering effective ethics education programs is vital for supporting the Bioethics Program's mission and vision. By creating engaging and interactive training sessions, utilizing advanced technologies, and continuously evaluating and improving educational content, the program can ensure that healthcare practitioners are prepared to navigate ethical challenges with confidence and competence. Integrating the core bioethical principles into every aspect of ethics education reinforces the commitment to patient autonomy, beneficence, nonmaleficence, and public justice, ultimately enhancing the quality and compassion of patient care.

***

For the designing and delivering of ethics education programs, several forms and templates can be useful to support the creation, delivery, and evaluation of effective ethics education sessions. The following tools can help ensure that training programs are engaging, interactive, and continuously improved based on participant feedback.

***

## 8.1 Training Session Planning Template

**Purpose**: To guide the development of engaging and effective ethics training sessions, ensuring that all key elements are covered.

**Session Title**: [Title of the Training Session]
**Date and Time**: [Date and Time of the Session]
**Target Audience**: [Description of the Audience (e.g., clinicians, administrators, students)]

**Learning Objectives**:

- List the specific learning objectives for the session (e.g., "Participants will understand the principles of informed consent").

**Content Overview**:

- Provide an outline of the session content, including key topics and concepts to be covered.

**Teaching Methods**:

- Identify the teaching methods to be used (e.g., lecture, case study, role-playing, group discussion).

**Interactive Activities**:

- Describe any interactive activities planned for the session (e.g., simulations, breakout groups, peer feedback).

**Case Studies/Scenarios**:

- Outline the case studies or scenarios that will be used, including any relevant details and ethical dilemmas.

**Multimedia Elements**:

- List any multimedia elements that will be incorporated (e.g., videos, podcasts, interactive online tools).

**Materials Needed**:

- List any materials or equipment needed for the session (e.g., handouts, projector, whiteboard).

**Assessment and Feedback**:

- Describe how participant learning will be assessed (e.g., quizzes, group presentations) and how feedback will be gathered (e.g., post-session surveys).

**Facilitator Notes**:

- Include any additional notes or tips for the facilitator to ensure the session runs smoothly.

***

## 8.2 Participant Feedback Form for Training Sessions

**Purpose**: To gather structured feedback from participants on the effectiveness and relevance of the ethics training session.

**Session Title**: [Title of the Training Session]
**Date**: [Date of the Session]
**Facilitator**: [Name of Facilitator]

**Relevance of Content**:

1. How relevant was the content of the training session to your role and responsibilities?
   - ☐ Highly Relevant
   - ☐ Moderately Relevant
   - ☐ Slightly Relevant
   - ☐ Not Relevant

**Engagement Level**:

2. How engaging did you find the training session?
   - ☐ Very Engaging
   - ☐ Somewhat Engaging
   - ☐ Neutral
   - ☐ Not Engaging

**Interactive Activities**:

3. How effective were the interactive activities (e.g., role-playing, case studies) in helping you understand the ethical issues?
   - ☐ Very Effective
   - ☐ Somewhat Effective
   - ☐ Neutral
   - ☐ Not Effective

**Clarity of Presentation**:

4. How clear and understandable was the presentation of the material?
   - ☐ Very Clear
   - ☐ Somewhat Clear
   - ☐ Neutral
   - ☐ Not Clear

**Overall Satisfaction**:

5. Overall, how satisfied were you with the training session?
   - ☐ Very Satisfied
   - ☐ Satisfied
   - ☐ Neutral
   - ☐ Dissatisfied

**Key Takeaways**:

6. What were the most important takeaways or lessons you gained from this session?

**Suggestions for Improvement**:

7. Do you have any suggestions for improving future training sessions?

**Additional Comments**:

8. Is there anything else you would like to share about your experience with this training session?

***

## 8.3 Case Study Analysis Worksheet

**Purpose**: To guide participants through the analysis of ethical case studies during training sessions.

**Case Title**: [Title of the Case Study]
**Date**: [Date of the Analysis]
**Participant Name**: [Name of Participant]

**Case Summary**:
- Provide a brief summary of the case, including key facts and ethical dilemmas.

**Ethical Issues**:
- Identify the primary ethical issues involved in the case (e.g., autonomy, beneficence, confidentiality).

**Stakeholder Perspectives**:
- List the perspectives of the key stakeholders (e.g., patient, family, healthcare team).

**Ethical Principles Applied**:
- Describe the ethical principles that are relevant to the case and how they apply.

**Possible Solutions**:
- Outline the potential solutions to the ethical dilemmas, considering the benefits and risks of each option.

**Recommended Course of Action**:
- Provide your recommendation for resolving the ethical issues, including the rationale behind your decision.

**Reflection**:
- Reflect on the case and your analysis. What did you learn from this exercise, and how might it apply to your practice?

***

## 8.4 Simulation Scenario Template

**Purpose**: To design realistic and relevant simulation scenarios for ethics training sessions, allowing participants to practice their skills in a controlled environment.

**Scenario Title**: [Title of the Scenario]
**Date**: [Date of the Simulation]
**Facilitator**: [Name of Facilitator]

**Objective**:

- State the primary learning objectives of the simulation (e.g., "Participants will practice making ethical decisions in end-of-life care").

**Scenario Overview**:

- Provide a brief description of the scenario, including the setting, characters, and ethical dilemmas involved.

**Roles**:

- List the roles to be played by participants (e.g., physician, nurse, patient, family member) and provide background information for each role.

**Key Ethical Issues**:

- Identify the key ethical issues that participants will need to address during the simulation.

**Instructions for Participants**:

- Provide clear instructions on how the simulation will be conducted, including any specific tasks or decisions that need to be made.

**Debriefing Questions**:

- List questions to guide the debriefing session after the simulation, encouraging reflection on the ethical issues and decision-making process (e.g., "What were the most challenging aspects of this scenario?").

**Assessment Criteria**:

- Describe how participants' performance will be assessed (e.g., communication skills, ethical reasoning, ability to work as a team).

***

## 8.5 Ethics Education Program Evaluation Form

**Purpose**: To evaluate the overall effectiveness of the ethics education program and gather feedback for ongoing improvement.

**Program Title**: [Title of the Education Program]
**Date**: [Date of the Program]
**Program Coordinator**: [Name of Program Coordinator]

**Program Relevance**:

1. How relevant was the ethics education program to your professional development and daily responsibilities?
   ☐ Highly Relevant
   ☐ Moderately Relevant
   ☐ Slightly Relevant
   ☐ Not Relevant

**Quality of Content**:

2. How would you rate the quality of the content presented in the program?
   ☐ Excellent
   ☐ Good
   ☐ Fair
   ☐ Poor

**Effectiveness of Teaching Methods**:

3. How effective were the teaching methods used in the program (e.g., lectures, workshops, simulations)?
   ☐ Very Effective
   ☐ Somewhat Effective
   ☐ Neutral
   ☐ Not Effective

**Impact on Practice**:

4. How has this program impacted your approach to ethical decision-making in your practice?
   - ☐ Significant Impact
   - ☐ Moderate Impact
   - ☐ Slight Impact
   - ☐ No Impact

**Areas for Improvement**:

5. What areas of the program could be improved in future iterations?

**Suggestions for Future Topics**:

6. Are there any specific topics you would like to see covered in future ethics education programs?

**Additional Comments**:

7. Please share any additional comments or feedback about the program.

***

## Further Readings and References


### Creating Engaging and Effective Training Sessions

- Knowles, M. S., Holton, E. F., & Swanson, R. A. (2011). The Adult Learner: The Definitive Classic in Adult Education and Human Resource Development (7th ed.). Butterworth-Heinemann.
  - *A definitive guide on adult learning principles and practices, offering insights into creating engaging and effective training sessions tailored to adult learners.*
- Silberman, M. (2015). Active Training: A Handbook of Techniques, Designs, Case Examples, and Tips (4th ed.). Wiley.
  - *Provides a comprehensive collection of techniques and tips for designing and delivering interactive and impactful training sessions, including practical case examples.*

### Using Interactive Workshops, Case Studies, and Simulations

- Brookfield, S. D., & Preskill, S. (2016). The Discussion Book: 50 Great Ways to Get People Talking. Jossey-Bass.
  - *Offers a variety of interactive discussion techniques and activities to foster engagement and participation in educational settings.*
- Kohn, L. T., Corrigan, J. M., & Donaldson, M. S. (Eds.). (2000). To Err Is Human: Building a Safer Health System. National Academy Press.
  - *Highlights the importance of patient safety and the role of interactive workshops, case studies, and simulations in improving healthcare practices and outcomes.*

### Evaluating and Improving Education Programs


- Kirkpatrick, D. L., & Kirkpatrick, J. D. (2006). Evaluating Training Programs: The Four Levels (3rd ed.). Berrett-Koehler Publishers.
  - *Introduces the Kirkpatrick Model for evaluating training programs, providing a comprehensive framework for assessing and improving educational initiatives.*
- Reeves, S., Perrier, L., Goldman, J., Freeth, D., & Zwarenstein, M. (2013). Interprofessional education: Effects on professional practice and healthcare outcomes (update). The Cochrane Database of Systematic Reviews, (3), CD002213.
  - *Reviews the impact of interprofessional education on professional practice and healthcare outcomes, offering insights into effective evaluation and improvement strategies.*


***

# Chapter 9: Outreach and Professional Engagement

Outreach and professional engagement are vital components of the Bioethics Program, enabling the dissemination of ethical principles and the development of a robust bioethical culture both within and beyond the healthcare institution. This chapter outlines strategies for providing ethics-related education and outreach, emphasizing the integration of the four core bioethical principles—patient autonomy (informed consent), practitioner beneficence (maximize benefits), practitioner nonmaleficence (minimize burdens), and public justice (ensure fairness). These activities aim to ensure compliance with institutional policies, established medical standards of care, and legal mandates, aligning with the Bioethics Program's mission and vision.

## Organizing Workshops, Seminars, and Conferences:

The Bioethics Program Director should organize and lead educational events that bring together healthcare professionals, ethics consultants, and other stakeholders to discuss ethical issues and share best practices. Key elements of these activities include:

- **Workshops and Seminars**: These events should focus on current ethical issues in healthcare, such as end-of-life decision-making, patient consent, and resource allocation. Workshops should be interactive, allowing participants to engage in discussions, case studies, and role-playing scenarios that highlight ethical dilemmas and the application of core bioethical principles.
- **Conferences**: Hosting or participating in conferences allows the Bioethics Program to reach a wider audience, including national and international bioethics communities. Conferences should include keynote presentations, panel discussions, and

breakout sessions that address diverse topics, such as emerging technologies, cultural competence in healthcare, and policy development.

- **Targeted Training Sessions**: Ethics-related training sessions should be tailored to the specific needs of various healthcare professionals. For example, training for clinicians might focus on informed consent and patient communication, while sessions for administrators might address policy development and ethical oversight.

## Collaborating with Other Bioethics Leaders

Collaboration with other bioethics leaders is essential for sharing knowledge and developing regional and national policies. The director should:

1. **Build Partnerships**: Establish partnerships with healthcare organizations, academic institutions, and professional organizations. Collaborative efforts might include joint research projects, shared training programs, and the development of ethics guidelines.
2. **Share Best Practices**: By working with other bioethics leaders, the director can exchange insights and strategies for addressing common ethical challenges. Regular meetings, both in-person and virtual, can facilitate ongoing dialogue and collaboration.
3. **Engage in Policy Development**: The director should actively participate in developing regional and national policies that promote ethical healthcare practices. This involves contributing to policy discussions, drafting guidelines, and advocating for standards that reflect the core bioethical principles.

## Promoting the Visibility and Impact of the Bioethics Program

Enhancing the visibility and impact of the Bioethics Program is crucial for establishing its reputation and influence. The director can achieve this by:

1. **Presenting at Conferences**: Regular presentations at professional conferences help promote the work of the Bioethics Program and position it as a leader in the field. Topics should reflect the program's expertise and address contemporary ethical issues.
2. **Publishing Articles and Papers**: Contributing to academic journals, professional newsletters, and other publications raises awareness of the program's work. Articles should highlight ethical challenges and offer solutions based on the core bioethical principles.
3. **Engaging with the Media**: By engaging with local and national media, the director can raise public awareness about important ethical issues in healthcare. Media engagement might include writing opinion pieces, giving interviews, and participating in public forums.

## Educating the General Public

Outreach programs aimed at educating the general public about bioethics can foster a broader understanding and appreciation of ethical issues in healthcare. Strategies include:

1. **Community Workshops**: Organizing workshops for community members on topics such as patient rights, end-of-life care, and healthcare decision-making can help educate the public about ethical considerations in healthcare.
2. **Educational Materials**: Creating pamphlets, brochures, and online resources that explain bioethical concepts in accessible language can provide valuable information to patients and their families.
3. **Engaging with Schools and Community Organizations**: Collaborating with schools to incorporate bioethics education into the curriculum and partnering with community organizations to offer educational programs can help promote ethical awareness at a grassroots level.

## Participating in Policy Discussions and Advocacy

The director should actively seek opportunities to participate in policy discussions and advocacy efforts related to bioethics. This can involve:

1. **Working with Government Agencies**: Engaging with local, state, and federal agencies to advocate for policies that promote ethical healthcare practices. This might include providing expert testimony, participating in advisory committees, and collaborating on policy development.
2. **Partnering with Professional Organizations**: Collaborating with organizations such as the American Society of Bioethics and Humanities (ASBH) and the Association of Bioethics Program Directors (ABPD) to influence policy and practice.
3. **Advocacy Efforts**: The director should support advocacy efforts that align with the core bioethical principles, such as promoting access to care, ensuring informed consent, and protecting patient rights.

## Engaging with Local, State, National, and International Communities

**Local and State Engagement**:

Engagement with local and state communities is essential for building a strong foundation for the Bioethics Program. The director should:

1. **Participate in Local Networks**: Join local ethics committees, healthcare coalitions, and professional associations to share expertise and build relationships. Local engagement helps address region-specific ethical issues and promotes ethical practices in the community.
2. **Collaborate with State Agencies**: Work with state health departments and regulatory bodies to develop and implement ethical guidelines and policies. This collaboration can ensure

that state-level healthcare practices align with core bioethical principles and legal requirements.

3. **Conduct Regional Workshops**: Organizing workshops at the state level can provide ethics education to a broader audience, including rural healthcare providers and community health organizations.

**National Engagement**:

Engaging with national bioethics communities helps the Bioethics Program stay informed about current developments and contribute to the broader field. The director should:

1. **Participate in National Conferences**: Attending and presenting at national conferences provides opportunities for learning, networking, and influencing the national bioethics agenda. Sessions should highlight the integration of ethical principles in clinical practice and policy development.
2. **Contribute to National Committees**: Serving on national committees and task forces allows the director to contribute to developing ethical guidelines, standards, and policies that impact healthcare practice nationwide.
3. **Collaborate on National Research Projects**: Engaging in national research projects related to bioethics can help advance the field and provide valuable insights into ethical challenges and solutions.

**International Engagement:**

Engaging with international bioethics organizations and initiatives broadens the Bioethics Program's perspective and influence. The director should:

1. **Attend International Conferences**: Participating in international conferences allows the Bioethics Program to learn from global best practices and contribute to the international discourse on bioethics.

2. **Collaborate on Global Initiatives**: Partnering with international organizations on research, policy development, and educational initiatives helps address global ethical challenges and promotes the exchange of knowledge and expertise.
3. **Contribute to International Ethical Guidelines**: The director should participate in developing international ethical guidelines and standards, ensuring that global healthcare practices reflect core bioethical principles.

### Building Networks and Collaborations

Building strong networks and collaborations is crucial for enhancing the impact of the Bioethics Program. The director should:

1. **Identify Key Stakeholders**: Engage with key stakeholders, including healthcare providers, academic institutions, government agencies, and non-governmental organizations, to establish collaborative partnerships.
2. **Develop Formal Agreements**: Create formal partnerships through Memorandums of Understanding (MOUs) or collaborative agreements that outline shared goals, responsibilities, and resources.
3. **Leverage Resources**: Collaborations allow the Bioethics Program to leverage resources, such as expertise, funding, and technology, to enhance its capacity to address ethical challenges.

### Engaging in Joint Research and Training Programs

Joint research and training programs can enhance the Bioethics Program's ability to address complex ethical issues. The director should:

1. **Initiate Collaborative Research Projects**: Collaborate with academic institutions and other organizations to conduct research on ethical issues in healthcare. Research topics might include patient consent processes, ethical decision-making in

end-of-life care, and the impact of emerging technologies on patient autonomy.

2. **Develop Shared Training Programs**: Partner with other healthcare organizations to develop and deliver ethics training programs. Joint training sessions can provide diverse perspectives and expertise, enriching the learning experience for participants.
3. **Promote Interdisciplinary Collaboration**: Encourage collaboration between healthcare professionals, ethicists, legal experts, and policymakers to address ethical issues from multiple perspectives.

## Promoting Visibility and Credibility

To enhance the Bioethics Program's visibility and credibility, the director should:

1. **Engage in Public Speaking**: Public speaking engagements, such as lectures, panel discussions, and community talks, raise awareness of the Bioethics Program and its work.
2. **Utilize Social Media and Online Platforms**: Engaging with audiences through social media and online platforms can extend the reach of the Bioethics Program. Sharing updates, resources, and insights on ethical issues can attract a wider audience and foster community engagement.
3. **Publish Regularly**: Regular publications in academic journals, professional magazines, and online blogs help establish the Bioethics Program as a thought leader in the field. Publications should address current ethical challenges and propose practical solutions.

## Conclusion

Outreach and professional engagement are critical for the success and influence of the Bioethics Program. By providing ethics-related education, engaging with local, state, national, and international communities, and building strong networks and collaborations, the program can promote ethical healthcare practices and contribute to the broader field of bioethics. Integrating the core bioethical principles into all outreach

***

For outreach and professional engagement, several forms and templates can be helpful to facilitate the planning, execution, and evaluation of ethics-related education, outreach, and professional engagement activities. The following tools will help ensure that the Bioethics Program Director's efforts are organized, impactful, and well-documented.

***

## 9.1 Outreach and Professional Engagement Planning Template

**Purpose**: To plan and organize ethics-related education and outreach activities, ensuring that all key elements are considered.

**Event/Activity Title**: [Title of the Event or Activity]
**Date and Time**: [Date and Time]
**Target Audience**: [Description of the Audience (e.g., healthcare professionals, students, public)]

**Objectives**:

- List the specific objectives of the outreach or engagement activity (e.g., "Increase awareness of bioethics in end-of-life care").

**Content Overview**:

- Provide an outline of the content or topics to be covered during the event or activity.

**Teaching/Engagement Methods**:

- Identify the methods to be used (e.g., lectures, workshops, panel discussions, webinars).

**Speakers/Facilitators**:

- List the names and titles of speakers or facilitators involved in the event.

**Materials Needed**:

- List any materials or equipment required (e.g., handouts, brochures, multimedia equipment).

**Promotion and Outreach**:

- Describe the strategies for promoting the event (e.g., social media, email newsletters, flyers).

**Partnerships and Collaborations**:

- Identify any collaborating organizations or partners involved in the event.

**Budget**:

- Outline the budget for the event, including costs for materials, speakers, venue, and promotion.

**Logistics**:

- Describe the logistics of the event, including venue, seating arrangements, and technical support.

**Evaluation Plan**:

- Describe how the success of the event will be evaluated (e.g., participant surveys, attendance metrics, post-event interviews).

**Follow-Up Actions**:

- List any follow-up actions required after the event, such as sending thank-you notes or distributing materials.

***

## 9.2 Participant Feedback Form for Outreach Events

**Purpose**: To gather feedback from participants on the effectiveness and impact of the ethics-related outreach event.

**Event Title**: [Title of the Event]
**Date**: [Date of the Event]

**Overall Satisfaction**:

1. How satisfied were you with the event overall?
   - ☐ Very Satisfied
   - ☐ Satisfied
   - ☐ Neutral
   - ☐ Dissatisfied

**Relevance of Content**:

2. How relevant was the content of the event to your interests or professional needs?
   - ☐ Highly Relevant
   - ☐ Moderately Relevant
   - ☐ Slightly Relevant
   - ☐ Not Relevant

**Speaker/Facilitator Effectiveness**:

3. How effective were the speakers/facilitators in delivering the content and engaging the audience?
   - ☐ Very Effective
   - ☐ Effective
   - ☐ Neutral
   - ☐ Ineffective

**Usefulness of Materials**:

4. How useful were the materials provided (e.g., handouts, slides, brochures)?
   - ☐ Very Useful
   - ☐ Useful
   - ☐ Neutral
   - ☐ Not Useful

**Impact on Understanding of Bioethics**:

5. How much did this event enhance your understanding of bioethics?
   - ☐ Significant Impact
   - ☐ Moderate Impact
   - ☐ Slight Impact
   - ☐ No Impact

**Suggestions for Improvement**:

6. What could be improved for future events?

**Additional Comments**:

7. Please share any additional comments or feedback about this event.

***

## 9.3 Networking and Collaboration Log

**Purpose**: To document and track networking and collaboration efforts with other organizations, including key contacts and outcomes.

**Date of Interaction**: [Date]
**Organization/Partner Name**: [Name of the Organization or Partner]
**Contact Person**: [Name, Title, and Contact Information]

**Type of Interaction**:
- ☐ Meeting
- ☐ Email Exchange
- ☐ Conference
- ☐ Workshop
- ☐ Joint Project
- ☐ *Other* [Specify]

**Summary of Discussion/Collaboration**:
- Briefly summarize the key points discussed and any agreements or actions decided.

**Follow-Up Actions**:
- List any follow-up actions required, including deadlines and responsible parties.

**Outcomes/Results**:
- Document any outcomes or results from the interaction (e.g., new partnerships, joint projects, shared resources).

**Next Steps**:
- Outline the next steps for continuing or expanding the collaboration.

***

## 9.4 Outreach Program Evaluation Template

**Purpose**: To evaluate the overall effectiveness of outreach programs and initiatives, ensuring continuous improvement.

**Program Title**: [Title of the Outreach Program]
**Date**: [Date of the Program]
**Program Coordinator**: [Name of Program Coordinator]

**Program Objectives**:
1. Were the objectives of the program met?
   - ☐ Fully Met
   - ☐ Partially Met
   - ☐ Not Met

**Participation Level**:
2. How would you rate the level of participation and engagement in the program?
   - ☐ High Participation
   - ☐ Moderate Participation
   - ☐ Low Participation

**Content Relevance and Quality**:
3. How relevant and high-quality was the content delivered in the program?
   - ☐ Excellent
   - ☐ Good
   - ☐ Fair
   - ☐ Poor

**Impact on Participants**:

4. What impact did the program have on participants' understanding or behavior regarding bioethics?
   - ☐ Significant Impact
   - ☐ Moderate Impact
   - ☐ Slight Impact
   - ☐ No Impact

**Promotion and Outreach Effectiveness**:

5. How effective were the promotion and outreach efforts in attracting participants?
   - ☐ Very Effective
   - ☐ Effective
   - ☐ Neutral
   - ☐ Ineffective

**Partnerships and Collaborations**:

6. How successful were the partnerships and collaborations in supporting the program?
   - ☐ Very Successful
   - ☐ Moderately Successful
   - ☐ Slightly Successful
   - ☐ Not Successful

**Areas for Improvement**:

7. What areas of the program could be improved in future iterations?

**Suggestions for Future Programs**:

8. Are there any specific topics or formats you would like to see in future outreach programs?

**Additional Comments**:

9. Please share any additional comments or feedback about the program.

***

## 9.5 Policy Advocacy Planning Template

**Purpose**: To organize and plan bioethics-related policy advocacy efforts, ensuring that objectives and strategies are clearly defined.

**Advocacy Issue**: [Description of the Policy or Ethical Issue]
**Date**: [Date of Planning]
**Advocacy Coordinator**: [Name of Advocacy Coordinator]

**Objective**:

- State the primary objective of the advocacy effort (e.g., "Influence state legislation on end-of-life care").

**Target Audience**:

- Identify the target audience(s) for the advocacy effort (e.g., policymakers, healthcare professionals, the general public).

**Key Messages**:

- Outline the key messages to be communicated during the advocacy effort.

**Strategies and Tactics**:

- Describe the strategies and tactics to be used (e.g., public speaking, writing op-eds, meeting with policymakers, organizing rallies).

**Partnerships and Collaborations**:

- Identify any partners or allies involved in the advocacy effort.

**Resources Needed**:

- List the resources required (e.g., funding, materials, volunteer support).

**Timeline**:

- Provide a timeline for the advocacy effort, including key milestones and deadlines.

**Evaluation Plan**:

- Describe how the success of the advocacy effort will be measured and evaluated.

**Follow-Up Actions**:

- List any follow-up actions required after the advocacy effort, such as debriefing sessions or continued engagement.

***

## Further Readings and References

### Providing Ethics-related Education and Outreach


- Callahan, D. (1999). The Role of the Ethicist. Hastings Center Report, 29(4), 32-39.
  - *Explores the multifaceted role of ethicists in education and outreach, emphasizing their contributions to public discourse and ethical awareness.*
- Singer, P. A., & Viens, A. M. (Eds.). (2008). The Cambridge Textbook of Bioethics. Cambridge University Press.
  - *A comprehensive reference on bioethics, covering key topics and issues relevant for providing ethics-related education and outreach.*


### Engaging with Local, State, National, and International Communities


- Lolas, F. (2010). Bioethics in international perspective. Acta Bioethica, 16(1), 9-15.
  - *Discusses the global dimensions of bioethics, highlighting the importance of engaging with communities at various levels to address ethical challenges.*
- Sugarman, J., & Sulmasy, D. P. (Eds.). (2010). Methods in Medical Ethics (2nd ed.). Georgetown University Press.
  - *Provides an overview of methodologies in medical ethics, emphasizing the significance of engaging with diverse communities to enhance ethical practices.*


### Building Networks and Collaborations


- Bryson, J. M. (2011). Strategic Planning for Public and Nonprofit Organizations: A Guide to Strengthening and Sustaining Organizational Achievement (4th ed.). Jossey-Bass.
  - *Offers a guide to strategic planning, focusing on building networks and collaborations to achieve organizational goals and sustain achievements.*

- Powell, W. W., & Grodal, S. (2005). Networks of innovators. In J. Fagerberg, D. C. Mowery, & R. R. Nelson (Eds.), The Oxford Handbook of Innovation (pp. 56-85). Oxford University Press.
  - *Examines the role of networks in fostering innovation, providing insights into building effective collaborations and partnerships in the field of bioethics.*


***

# Review Questions

**True/False Questions:**

1. Active listening involves giving full attention to the speaker, asking clarifying questions, and reflecting back what has been said to ensure understanding.
True or False?

2. Empathetic engagement in ethics consultations means responding with compassion and support, recognizing and validating the emotions and experiences of others.
True or False?

3. It is unnecessary for a Bioethics Program Director to stay informed about the latest developments in bioethics and healthcare law.
True or False?

4. Effective mediation during ethics consultations requires the ability to remain neutral and objective.
True or False?

5. Providing balanced ethical advice means considering only the benefits of different options.
True or False?

**Multiple-Choice Questions:**

6. Which of the following is a crucial element for effective ethics consultations?
a) Ignoring the perspectives of patients and families
b) Gathering and considering all relevant information
c) Avoiding documentation of consultation outcomes
d) Restricting input to only medical professionals

7. What should be included in an ethics consultation to ensure clarity and balance?
a) Jargon and technical language
b) Unilateral decisions without stakeholder input
c) Thorough analysis of ethical dimensions and clear communication
d) Ignoring the risks of different options

**Clinical Vignettes:**

8. During an ethics consultation, a patient's family is in conflict with the healthcare team about continuing life-sustaining treatment. What is the best course of action for the Bioethics Program Director?
a) Ignore the family's concerns
b) Facilitate a meeting to mediate the discussion and explore potential solutions
c) Side with the healthcare team without discussion
d) Recommend the family seek legal action

9. A nurse reports that a physician consistently avoids informing patients about alternative treatments. What should the Bioethics Program Director do?
a) Tell the nurse to follow the physician's orders
b) Review the situation and discuss the ethical implications with the healthcare team
c) Ignore the concern
d) Advise the nurse to find another job

10. A patient expresses concerns about the potential discrimination and privacy issues related to a new genetic testing policy. What should the Bioethics Program Director do?
a) Dismiss the patient's concerns as unfounded
b) Explain the ethical implications and privacy measures in place
c) Suggest the patient avoid genetic testing altogether
d) Recommend the patient consult a lawyer

## Correct Answers:

1. True
2. True
3. False (It is necessary for a Bioethics Program Director to stay informed about the latest developments in bioethics and healthcare law.)
4. True
5. False (Providing balanced ethical advice means considering both the benefits and the risks of different options.)
6. b) Gathering and considering all relevant information
7. c) Thorough analysis of ethical dimensions and clear communication
8. b) Facilitate a meeting to mediate the discussion and explore potential solutions
9. b) Review the situation and discuss the ethical implications with the healthcare team
10. b) Explain the ethical implications and privacy measures in place

***

# Part IV: Leveraging Technology for Bioethics

## Chapter 10: Integrating Ethics into Electronic Health Records (EHR)

Integrating ethical considerations into Electronic Health Records (EHR) is critical for supporting the Bioethics Program's mission to provide comprehensive ethics consultation, education, and policy development. By embedding ethical documentation practices into EHR systems, healthcare providers can ensure that ethical principles—patient autonomy (informed consent), practitioner beneficence (maximize benefits), practitioner nonmaleficence (minimize burdens), and public justice (ensure fairness)—are consistently upheld. This chapter discusses strategies for leveraging EHR systems to enhance ethical documentation, promote transparency and accountability, and support high-quality, ethical patient care.

### Utilizing the EHR System for Ethical Documentation

**EHR Systems in Use**:

Major EHR systems widely used in American hospitals include Epic Systems, Cerner, MEDITECH, Allscripts, Athenahealth, McKesson, NextGen Healthcare, and eClinicalWorks. These systems provide robust platforms for documenting patient care and can be tailored to include ethical considerations. Effective use of these systems for ethical documentation involves:

1. **Customizing EHR for Ethical Needs**: The director should collaborate with IT professionals and EHR administrators to customize the system for ethical documentation. This customization might include creating fields for ethics consultations, developing templates for informed consent, and

integrating ethical decision-making frameworks. Customization ensures that ethical considerations are seamlessly integrated into clinical workflows.

2. **Training Practitioners**: Comprehensive training is essential for ensuring that healthcare providers can use EHR systems effectively for ethical documentation. Training should cover technical aspects of the EHR, ethical principles, and practical application. Role-playing scenarios and case studies can help practitioners learn to document ethical issues accurately and consistently.
3. **Developing Guidelines and Templates**: The director should develop standardized guidelines and templates for ethical documentation within the EHR. These templates might include prompts for documenting informed consent, noting ethical concerns, and outlining the ethical analysis and recommendations. Standardization helps ensure consistency and completeness in documentation.
4. **Implementing Regular Audits**: To maintain high standards of ethical documentation, regular audits should be conducted. Audits can help identify discrepancies, ensure compliance with ethical standards, and provide feedback for continuous improvement. The director should establish a protocol for auditing ethical documentation and addressing any issues identified.

### Promoting the Use of EHR for Ethical Decision-Making

Awareness campaigns and internal communication strategies can promote the benefits and importance of using EHR systems for ethical documentation. The director can:

1. **Highlight Success Stories**: Share examples of cases where the EHR facilitated ethical decision-making and improved patient care. Success stories can motivate practitioners to engage more deeply with ethical documentation practices.

2. **Recognize Excellence**: Acknowledge and reward practitioners who demonstrate excellence in ethical documentation. Recognition can reinforce the importance of ethical practices and encourage others to follow suit.
3. **Facilitate Ongoing Support**: Provide continuous support and resources for practitioners, including refresher courses and a help desk for EHR-related queries. Ensuring that practitioners have access to support can enhance their confidence and proficiency in using the EHR for ethical documentation.

## Best Practices for Using SOAP Notes in Ethics Consultation

SOAP Notes (Subjective, Objective, Assessment, Plan) are a standardized method for documenting ethics consultations. They provide a clear, structured approach to capturing all relevant information, supporting effective communication and decision-making. The director should ensure that SOAP Notes are used consistently across all ethics consultations by:

1. **Training Practitioners**: Training should focus on how to use SOAP Notes effectively. Practitioners need to be skilled in capturing the patient's narrative (Subjective), documenting clinical findings and observations (Objective), conducting ethical analysis (Assessment), and outlining planned actions (Plan). Training should include real-world examples and scenarios that practitioners might encounter.
2. **Providing Templates**: Standardized templates for SOAP Notes can guide practitioners in documenting consultations comprehensively and accurately. Templates should include prompts that encourage practitioners to consider all relevant aspects of the consultation, including patient autonomy, beneficence, nonmaleficence, and justice.
3. **Encouraging Reflection**: Regular team meetings and debriefings should include discussions on the use of SOAP Notes. Practitioners should reflect on their experiences, share

insights, and provide feedback to one another. This ongoing dialogue can help improve the use of SOAP Notes and enhance the quality of ethics consultations.

## Integrating SOAP Notes Across Clinical Practice

To promote thorough and precise documentation throughout clinical practice, the director should encourage the use of SOAP Notes beyond ethics consultations. This approach can:

1. **Standardize Documentation**: By using SOAP Notes consistently, practitioners can develop a habit of detailed documentation, improving overall communication and patient care.
2. **Facilitate Interdisciplinary Communication**: SOAP Notes provide a clear and structured format that can be easily understood by all members of the healthcare team. This consistency supports interdisciplinary communication and ensures that all team members are informed about the ethical dimensions of patient care.
3. **Support Continuous Improvement**: Regular workshops and training sessions on SOAP Notes can reinforce their importance and provide opportunities for practitioners to refine their skills. Continuous improvement in documentation practices supports high standards of patient care and ethical decision-making.

## Ensuring Transparency and Accountability in EHR

Transparency in ethical documentation is essential for building trust and ensuring that ethical considerations are consistently applied. The director should:

1. **Create Clear Guidelines**: Develop clear and comprehensive guidelines for ethical documentation. These guidelines should outline the expectations for documenting ethics consultations, informed consent, and other ethical considerations.
2. **Ensure Accessibility**: Ethical documentation should be accessible to all relevant stakeholders, including healthcare

providers, patients, and, when appropriate, family members. Accessibility supports transparency and enables informed decision-making.

3. **Educate Patients**: Patients should be informed about their rights and how their ethical concerns are documented and addressed. Providing patients with clear and accessible information can enhance their trust in the healthcare system and encourage open communication about ethical issues.

## Implementing Regular Audits and Reviews

Regular audits and reviews are crucial for maintaining the integrity of ethical documentation. The director should:

1. **Conduct Routine Audits**: Establish a schedule for routine audits of ethical documentation within the EHR. Audits should assess compliance with ethical standards, accuracy of documentation, and adherence to guidelines.
2. **Provide Feedback**: Use audit findings to provide constructive feedback to practitioners. Feedback should highlight areas of strength and identify opportunities for improvement. The goal is to support continuous learning and enhancement of ethical documentation practices.
3. **Address Non-Compliance**: Develop protocols for addressing instances of non-compliance with ethical documentation standards. This might involve additional training, changes to documentation processes, or other corrective actions.

## Leveraging Technology for Enhanced Transparency

Technology can play a key role in promoting transparency and accountability. The director should:

1. **Use Secure Systems**: Ensure that the EHR system is secure and protects patient privacy while allowing authorized access to ethical documentation. Security measures should comply with relevant legal and regulatory requirements.

2. **Implement Automated Alerts**: Automated alerts can remind practitioners of follow-up actions or ethical considerations that need attention. Alerts can help ensure that ethical issues are addressed promptly and consistently.
3. **Utilize Dashboards and Reports**: Develop dashboards and reports that track key metrics related to ethical documentation. These tools can provide insights into trends, highlight areas for improvement, and support data-driven decision-making.

**Conclusion**

Integrating ethics into Electronic Health Records is essential for supporting the Bioethics Program's mission and ensuring that ethical principles are consistently applied in patient care. By utilizing EHR systems for ethical documentation, promoting the use of SOAP Notes, and ensuring transparency and accountability, the program can enhance the accuracy, accessibility, and effectiveness of ethical decision-making. Leveraging technology to support ethical practices reinforces the commitment to patient autonomy, beneficence, nonmaleficence, and public justice, ultimately contributing to high-quality, compassionate patient care.

***

The following templates are designed to support the integration of ethical considerations into the EHR system, ensuring that all relevant information is documented accurately and consistently. By providing structured tools and training, the Bioethics Program Director can enhance the quality of ethical documentation and support effective decision-making across the organization.

***

## 10.1 EHR Ethical Documentation Customization Request Form

**Purpose**: To request customization of the EHR system to include specific fields and templates for ethical documentation.

**Date**: [Date]
**Requested by**: [Name/Title]
**Department**: [Department Name]
**Contact Information**: [Phone Number, Email Address]

Customization Details

- **Purpose of Customization**:
  [Explain the need for customization, e.g., to document ethics consultations, informed consent, etc.]
- **Specific Fields Required**:
  [List the specific fields or sections to be added, e.g., "Ethics Consultation Summary," "Informed Consent Details."]
- **Templates to be Developed**:
  [Describe any templates needed, e.g., "SOAP note template for ethics consultations."]
- **Integration with Existing Systems**:
  [Detail how the customization should integrate with other EHR functionalities.]

Expected Outcomes

- **Benefits of Customization**:
  [Describe the expected benefits, e.g., improved accuracy in ethical documentation, better support for ethical decision-making.]
- **Potential Challenges**:
  [List any potential challenges or concerns, e.g., user training needs, impact on workflow.]

**Requested Implementation Date**: [Date]
**Approved by**: [Name/Title]
**Date of Approval**: [Date]

Follow-up and Evaluation

- **Post-Implementation Review Date**: [Date]
- **Feedback Mechanism**: [Describe how feedback will be collected and evaluated.]

***

## 10.2 SOAP Notes EHR Integration

**Purpose:** To ensure the effective integration of SOAP Notes into the Electronic Health Records (EHR) system, enhancing documentation practices, compliance, and patient care.

**1. Customization of EHR Templates**

☐ Create SOAP Note Templates:

- Ensure all necessary fields for Subjective, Objective, Assessment, and Plan components are included.
- Use drop-down menus, checkboxes, and text fields to standardize data entry.

☐ Standardize Data Entry:

- Implement consistent input processes across all user interfaces.

**2. Training and Education**

☐ User Training:

- Train healthcare providers on using the SOAP note template within the EHR system.

☐ Best Practices:

- Provide guidelines emphasizing clarity, accuracy, and adherence to legal and institutional standards.

**3. Integration with Patient Records**

☐ Link SOAP Notes to Patient Records:

- Ensure automatic linkage of SOAP Notes to the patient's electronic health record.

☐ Cross-Reference Documentation:

- Enable cross-referencing with consent forms, lab results, and previous treatment plans.

**4. Compliance and Security**

- ☐ HIPAA Compliance:
  - Confirm that the EHR system is compliant with HIPAA and other relevant privacy laws.
- ☐ Audit Trails:
  - Implement audit trails to monitor access and changes to SOAP Notes within the EHR.

**5. Automation and Alerts**

- ☐ Automated Reminders:
  - Set up reminders for follow-up actions as documented in the Plan section.
- ☐ Alerts for Incomplete Documentation:
  - Implement alerts to ensure all sections of SOAP Notes are completed before finalizing the record.

**6. Continuous Improvement**

- ☐ Feedback Mechanism:
  - Incorporate a system for clinicians to report issues or suggest improvements to the SOAP note templates.
- ☐ Regular Updates:
  - Periodically review and update SOAP note templates to align with current clinical guidelines and policies.

**7. Interoperability**

- ☐ Integration with Other Systems:
  - Ensure the EHR system can share SOAP Notes across different platforms or institutions.
- ☐ Standardization Across Systems:
  - Work towards adopting standardized formats for use across different EHR systems.

**Completion:**

- ☐ Ensure all items on this checklist have been reviewed and addressed before finalizing the integration of SOAP Notes into the EHR.

***

## 10.3 EHR Ethical Documentation Audit Checklist

**Purpose**: To ensure the accuracy, consistency, and compliance of ethical documentation within the EHR system.

**Date of Audit**: [Date]
**Auditor**: [Name/Title]
**Department**: [Department Name]

**Documentation Completeness**

- ☐ All relevant fields are completed.
- ☐ Ethics consultation notes are recorded using the SOAP format.
- ☐ Informed consent documentation is present and complete.

**Ethical Analysis and Recommendations**

- ☐ Ethical issues are clearly identified and analyzed.
- ☐ Recommendations are based on established bioethical principles.
- ☐ Alternatives are discussed where applicable.

**Compliance with Standards**

- ☐ Documentation adheres to medical healthcare standards.
- ☐ Entries are compliant with institutional policies.
- ☐ Legal requirements are met in the documentation.

**Transparency and Accessibility**

- ☐ Documentation is clear and easily accessible to authorized personnel.
- ☐ Patient's perspective is documented and respected.
- ☐ All stakeholders are informed of the documentation outcomes.

**Follow-up and Implementation**

- ☐ Action steps are clearly outlined and assigned.
- ☐ Follow-up actions are documented and tracked.
- ☐ Any issues identified during the audit are addressed.

**Audit Findings**

- **Summary of Findings**:
  [Provide a brief summary of the audit findings.]
- **Recommendations for Improvement**:
  [List any recommendations for improving documentation practices.]

**Reviewed by**: [Name/Title]
**Date of Review**: [Date]

**Follow-up Actions**: [Describe any follow-up actions required.]

***

## 10.4 EHR Ethical Documentation Training Agenda

---

**Purpose**: To outline the content and structure of training sessions on the use of EHR for ethical documentation.

**Training Date**: [Date]
**Facilitator**: [Name/Title]
**Location**: [Location/Online Platform]

**Introduction and Overview**

- **Purpose of Training**
  [Brief introduction to the training session's objectives.]
- **Importance of Ethical Documentation**
  [Discuss the role of ethical documentation in patient care and decision-making.]

**Overview of EHR System**

- **Introduction to EHR Features**
  [Overview of relevant EHR features for ethical documentation.]
- **Customization for Ethical Documentation**
  [Discuss specific customizations made to the EHR for ethical purposes.]

**Using SOAP Notes in EHR**

- **Introduction to SOAP Notes**
  [Explanation of the SOAP format and its importance in ethics consultations.]
- **Practical Demonstration**
  [Live demonstration of how to complete SOAP Notes in the EHR system.]

**Hands-On Practice**

- **Interactive Exercise**
  [Participants practice documenting an ethics consultation using the SOAP format.]
- **Group Feedback**
  [Group discussion and feedback on the exercise.]

**Reviewing and Auditing Documentation**

- **Introduction to Audit Procedures**
  [Overview of the audit process for ethical documentation.]
- **Common Documentation Issues**
  [Discussion of common errors and how to avoid them.]

**Q&A and Wrap-Up**

- **Open Q&A Session**
  [Participants ask questions and seek clarification on any training content.]
- **Summary and Next Steps**
  [Recap key points and outline any follow-up actions or additional resources.]

***

## Further Readings and References

### Utilizing the EHR System for Ethical Documentation

- Glaser, J. P., & Salzberg, C. A. (2011). The Strategic Application of Information Technology in Health Care Organizations (3rd ed.). Jossey-Bass.
    - *Discusses strategic approaches to implementing information technology in healthcare, including the use of EHR systems for ethical documentation.*
- McGowan, J. J., & Berner, E. S. (Eds.). (2021). Health Informatics: An Interprofessional Approach (2nd ed.). Elsevier.
    - *Offers a comprehensive overview of health informatics, focusing on interprofessional approaches and the integration of ethics into EHR systems.*

### Best Practices for Using SOAP Notes in Ethics Consultation

- Bickley, L. S. (2017). Bates' Guide to Physical Examination and History Taking (12th ed.). Wolters Kluwer.
    - *Provides detailed guidance on using SOAP Notes effectively in clinical settings, including their application in ethics consultations.*
- Pomerantz, W. J., & Schafermeyer, R. (2002). SOAP documentation. Emergency Medicine Clinics of North America, 20(1), 165-174.
    - *Examines the principles and best practices of SOAP documentation, emphasizing their importance in maintaining accurate and ethical records in healthcare.*

### Ensuring Transparency and Accountability in EHR

- Kuhn, K. A., Warren, J. R., & Leong, T. Y. (Eds.). (2013). Informatics and Medicine: From Molecules to Populations. Springer.
    - *Explores the role of informatics in healthcare, highlighting the importance of transparency and accountability in EHR systems to ensure ethical standards.*

- Terry, N. P. (2013). Information technology's failure to disrupt healthcare. Nevada Law Journal, 13(3), 722-760.
    - *Analyzes the challenges and failures of information technology in transforming healthcare, stressing the need for ethical considerations and accountability in EHR implementation.*

***

# Chapter 11: Using Technology to Enhance Ethics Programs

The integration of digital tools and technology into ethics programs offers unprecedented opportunities to enhance ethical decision-making, education, and documentation. Leveraging these technologies aligns with the Bioethics Program's mission to uphold patient autonomy (informed consent), practitioner beneficence (maximize benefits), practitioner nonmaleficence (minimize burdens), and public justice (ensure fairness). This chapter explores how digital tools, data analytics, and emerging technologies can be effectively used to strengthen ethics programs, ensuring compliance with institutional policies, established medical standards of care, and legal mandates.

## Implementing Digital Tools for Ethics Rounds and Training

The use of online platforms and video conferencing tools can transform traditional ethics rounds into flexible and accessible virtual sessions. By creating virtual ethics rounds, the director can:

1. **Facilitate Broader Participation**: Allow practitioners to participate from remote locations, ensuring that ethical discussions and training sessions are inclusive and accessible. This flexibility supports engagement across various departments and shifts, promoting a culture of continuous ethical reflection and dialogue.

2. **Enhance Case Reviews**: Use virtual tools to present real-time case reviews, where practitioners can discuss and analyze ethical dilemmas. Digital tools can also facilitate the sharing of case documentation, multimedia content, and interactive elements, enriching the learning experience.

3. **Develop Online Training Modules**: Create comprehensive online training modules that include video lectures, interactive scenarios, quizzes, and discussion forums. These modules should cover core ethical principles, informed consent, and case-based learning. Online training enables practitioners to learn at their own pace and revisit materials as needed.
4. **Record Sessions for Future Reference**: Video conferencing platforms allow ethics rounds and training sessions to be recorded and archived. These recordings can serve as valuable resources for future training, continuous learning, and review by those who could not attend live sessions.

## Promoting Digital Tool Usage

To maximize the impact of digital tools in ethics programs, the director should:

1. **Create Awareness Campaigns**: Launch initiatives to educate practitioners about the availability and benefits of digital ethics tools. Highlight how these tools can enhance their practice and contribute to ethical decision-making.
2. **Provide Regular Training and Support**: Offer training sessions on using digital platforms effectively for ethics rounds and consultations. Continuous support should be available to address technical issues and help practitioners integrate digital tools into their daily routines.
3. **Recognize and Celebrate Ethical Behavior**: Recognize practitioners who effectively utilize digital tools in ethics consultations and training. Celebrating these efforts can motivate others to engage with these technologies, reinforcing a culture of ethical practice.

## Enhancing Collaboration with Digital Tools

Digital tools can significantly enhance collaboration among ethics committees and other stakeholders. The director should explore:

1. **Collaborative Platforms**: Use platforms that facilitate document sharing, asynchronous communication, and task tracking. Such tools allow for efficient coordination of ethics consultations and ensure that all relevant information is accessible to team members.
2. **Real-Time Communication**: Implement tools that allow for real-time discussions and decision-making among ethics committee members, even when they are not physically present. These tools can include secure messaging apps, chat rooms, and video calls.
3. **Mobile Applications**: Develop or adopt mobile applications that provide access to ethics resources, case studies, and decision-making frameworks. Mobile apps support on-the-go learning and enable practitioners to access information when needed, enhancing their ability to respond to ethical dilemmas.

## Leveraging Data Analytics for Ethics Quality Improvement

Data analytics can provide critical insights into the effectiveness of the Bioethics Program. The director should collaborate with data analysts and IT teams to:

1. **Develop Metrics and Dashboards**: Create dashboards that track key metrics related to ethics consultations, training activities, and policy implementation. Metrics might include the number of consultations, types of ethical issues addressed, time to resolution, and outcomes of ethical decisions.
2. **Analyze Trends in Ethical Issues**: Regular analysis of data can help identify trends and recurring ethical challenges. Understanding these trends allows the Bioethics Program to proactively address issues, tailor training programs, and refine policies.
3. **Evaluate Training Program Impact**: Use data to assess the effectiveness of ethics training programs. Metrics such as pre- and post-training knowledge assessments, participant feedback,

and behavioral changes can provide valuable insights into the impact of training.

## Promoting Data-Driven Ethics Quality Improvement

The director should ensure that data analytics is an integral part of the Bioethics Program by:

1. **Conducting Awareness and Training Sessions**: Educate practitioners on how data analytics can enhance ethics quality improvement. Training should focus on understanding and interpreting data, using dashboards, and making data-informed decisions.
2. **Encouraging a Culture of Data Literacy**: Foster a culture where practitioners value and use data to guide ethical decision-making. Regular workshops and discussions on the role of data in ethics can reinforce its importance.
3. **Utilizing Predictive Analytics**: Predictive analytics can identify potential ethical issues before they escalate. By analyzing patterns and data trends, the director can implement preventive measures and interventions, reducing ethical conflicts and enhancing patient care.

## Ensuring Accessibility and User-Friendliness

To maximize the benefits of data analytics, tools must be user-friendly. The director should:

1. **Simplify Data Presentation**: Ensure that data dashboards and reports are intuitive and easily understood by all stakeholders. Simplifying data presentation enhances usability and enables practitioners to quickly interpret and act on the information.
2. **Provide Continuous Training**: Offer ongoing training to develop data literacy skills among practitioners. This training should cover how to access, interpret, and use data effectively in their practice.

## Exploring Future Trends in Bioethics Technology

The bioethics field is rapidly evolving, with new technologies continually emerging. The director should:

1. **Investigate Artificial Intelligence (AI)**: AI can be used to analyze large volumes of ethical data, identify patterns, and support decision-making. The director should explore how AI can assist in ethical analysis and the documentation of complex cases.
2. **Explore Blockchain for Secure Documentation**: Blockchain technology offers secure, transparent, and tamper-proof documentation solutions. Its application in ethical documentation can ensure the integrity and confidentiality of sensitive information.
3. **Engage with Emerging Medical Technologies**: As new medical technologies emerge, they bring new ethical challenges. The director should stay informed about these advancements and ensure that the Bioethics Program is prepared to address their ethical implications.

## Fostering a Culture of Innovation and Continuous Improvement

Innovation is key to the success of the Bioethics Program. The director should:

1. **Create Opportunities for Experimentation**: Encourage practitioners to experiment with new technologies and approaches to ethical decision-making. Pilot projects and sandbox environments can provide safe spaces for innovation.
2. **Promote Continuous Learning**: Regularly offer workshops, seminars, and training on the latest technological advancements and their ethical implications. Keeping practitioners informed and engaged with new technologies supports a dynamic and responsive Bioethics Program.

3. **Collaborate with Technologists**: Build partnerships with technology developers and researchers to integrate ethical considerations into the design of new technologies. Collaboration ensures that ethical principles are embedded in technological solutions from the outset.

## Addressing Ethical Implications of Emerging Technologies

As new technologies are developed, they may pose ethical challenges. The director should:

1. **Engage in Ongoing Ethical Discussions**: Facilitate discussions on the ethical implications of emerging technologies within the Bioethics Program. These discussions can help anticipate and address potential ethical issues before they become problematic.
2. **Develop Guidelines and Policies**: Create guidelines and policies that address the ethical use of emerging technologies. Clear policies can provide direction and support for practitioners as they navigate new ethical landscapes.
3. **Stay Informed and Connected**: Attend conferences, participate in professional organizations, and engage with the broader bioethics community to stay informed about technological advancements and ethical considerations. Being connected to the field ensures that the Bioethics Program remains relevant and effective.

### Conclusion

Leveraging technology is essential for enhancing the Bioethics Program's capacity to uphold ethical principles and deliver high-quality patient care. By integrating digital tools into ethics rounds and training, utilizing data analytics for quality improvement, and exploring future technological trends, the program can remain innovative and responsive to the evolving needs of healthcare. These efforts align with the Bioethics Program's mission to promote patient autonomy, beneficence, nonmaleficence, and public justice, ensuring that ethical considerations are at the forefront of patient care and decision-making.

***

The Following templates are designed to support the integration of digital tools, data analytics, and emerging technologies into the Bioethics Program, ensuring that the program remains innovative, effective, and aligned with ethical standards. By providing structured tools and processes, the Bioethics Program Director can enhance the program's overall effectiveness and support high-quality, ethical patient care.

***

## 11.1 Digital Tools Implementation Plan

**Purpose**: To outline the plan for implementing digital tools to enhance ethics rounds and training programs.

**Date**: [Date]
**Prepared by**: [Name/Title]
**Department**: [Department Name]

**Objective**

- **Purpose of Implementation**:
  [Explain the goals of integrating digital tools into ethics rounds and training, e.g., improving accessibility, enhancing collaboration.]

**Digital Tools Selection**

- **Platforms/Tools Identified**:
  [List the specific digital tools and platforms to be used, e.g., Zoom for video conferencing, Moodle for online training.]
- **Features and Capabilities**:
  [Describe the key features of each tool and how they will be utilized in the Bioethics Program.]

**Implementation Steps**

- **Preparation**:
  [Outline the steps needed to prepare for implementation, such as setting up accounts, configuring tools, and creating content.]
- **Training**:
  [Describe the training plan for practitioners, including scheduled sessions, materials, and resources.]
- **Launch**:
  [Detail the timeline for launching the digital tools, including key milestones and deadlines.]

**Evaluation and Feedback**

- **Monitoring Usage and Effectiveness**:
  [Explain how the usage and effectiveness of the digital tools will be monitored, e.g., usage statistics, participant feedback.]
- **Continuous Improvement**:
  [Describe the process for gathering feedback and making improvements to the digital tools and their implementation.]

**Responsibilities**

- **Team Members Involved**:
  [List the individuals responsible for different aspects of the implementation, including IT support, training, and evaluation.]
- **Roles and Responsibilities**:
  [Define the roles and responsibilities of each team member.]

**Budget Considerations**

- **Estimated Costs**:
  [Provide an estimate of the costs associated with the implementation, including software licenses, training, and support.]
- **Funding Sources**:
  [Identify potential sources of funding, such as departmental budgets or grants.]

***

## 11.2 Data Analytics Metrics and Dashboard Development Guide

**Purpose**: To guide the development of metrics and dashboards for monitoring ethics consultations and training activities.

**Date**: [Date]
**Prepared by**: [Name/Title]
**Department**: [Department Name]

**Objective**

- **Purpose of Data Analytics**:
  [Explain the goals of using data analytics in the Bioethics Program, e.g., improving consultation outcomes, enhancing training effectiveness.]

**Key Metrics**

- **Consultation Metrics**:
  [List the key metrics to track for ethics consultations, e.g., number of consultations, response times, resolution rates.]
- **Training Metrics**:
  [List the key metrics to track for training activities, e.g., participation rates, completion rates, participant satisfaction.]

**Dashboard Design**

- **Dashboard Components**:
  [Describe the key components of the dashboard, such as graphs, tables, and charts.]
- **Data Sources**:
  [Identify the sources of data to be used in the dashboard, such as EHR systems, survey results, and training records.]

**Implementation Steps**

- **Data Integration**:
  [Outline the steps needed to integrate data from various sources into the dashboard.]
- **Dashboard Development**:
  [Detail the timeline for developing the dashboard, including key milestones and deadlines.]

**Evaluation and Feedback**

- **Monitoring Effectiveness**:
  [Explain how the effectiveness of the dashboard will be monitored, e.g., user feedback, accuracy of data.]
- **Continuous Improvement**:
  [Describe the process for gathering feedback and making improvements to the dashboard.]

**Responsibilities**

- **Team Members Involved**:
  [List the individuals responsible for different aspects of the dashboard development, including data analysts, IT support, and Bioethics Program staff.]
- **Roles and Responsibilities**:
  [Define the roles and responsibilities of each team member.]

**Budget Considerations**

- **Estimated Costs**:
  [Provide an estimate of the costs associated with the development and maintenance of the dashboard.]
- **Funding Sources**:
  [Identify potential sources of funding, such as departmental budgets or grants.]

***

## 11.3 Emerging Technology Exploration Template

**Purpose**: To explore and assess new technologies for potential integration into the Bioethics Program.

**Date**: [Date]
**Prepared by**: [Name/Title]
**Department**: [Department Name]

**Technology Overview**

- **Technology Name**:
  [Identify the technology being explored, e.g., Artificial Intelligence (AI), Blockchain.]
- **Description**:
  [Provide a brief description of the technology and its potential applications in bioethics.]

**Ethical Implications**

- **Potential Benefits**:
  [Describe the potential ethical benefits of the technology, e.g., enhanced decision-making, improved transparency.]
- **Potential Risks**:
  [Identify any ethical risks or concerns associated with the technology, e.g., privacy issues, bias in AI algorithms.]

**Feasibility Assessment**

- **Technical Feasibility**:
  [Evaluate the technical feasibility of implementing the technology within the Bioethics Program.]
- **Resource Requirements**:
  [Estimate the resources needed for implementation, including time, budget, and personnel.]

**Pilot Program Proposal**

- **Pilot Objectives**:
  [Define the objectives of a pilot program to test the technology in a controlled environment.]
- **Implementation Plan**:
  [Outline the steps needed to implement the pilot program, including key milestones and deadlines.]

**Evaluation and Feedback**

- **Monitoring and Evaluation**:
  [Describe how the pilot program will be monitored and evaluated, including metrics for success.]
- **Feedback Mechanism**:
  [Explain how feedback will be gathered from participants and stakeholders.]

**Recommendations**

- **Next Steps**:
  [Based on the findings, provide recommendations for whether and how to proceed with full-scale implementation.]

**Responsibilities**

- **Team Members Involved**:
  [List the individuals responsible for exploring the technology, conducting the pilot, and evaluating the results.]
- **Roles and Responsibilities**:
  [Define the roles and responsibilities of each team member.]

**Budget Considerations**

- **Estimated Costs**:
  [Provide an estimate of the costs associated with the pilot program and potential full-scale implementation.]
- **Funding Sources**:
  [Identify potential sources of funding, such as departmental budgets or grants.]

***

## Further Readings and References

### Implementing Digital Tools for Ethics Rounds and Training


- Hebda, T., Hunter, K., & Czar, P. (2019). Handbook of Informatics for Nurses & Healthcare Professionals (6th ed.). Pearson.
  - *A practical guide to informatics for healthcare professionals, including the use of digital tools to enhance ethics rounds and training programs.*
- Sanders, J. L., & Schneider, J. K. (2017). Ethical considerations of electronic communication in the era of HIPAA. Journal of the American Association of Nurse Practitioners, 29(2), 66-71.
  - *Discusses the ethical implications of electronic communication in healthcare, particularly in relation to HIPAA regulations and patient privacy.*


### Leveraging Data Analytics for Ethics Quality Improvement


- Raghupathi, W., & Raghupathi, V. (2014). Big data analytics in healthcare: Promise and potential. Health Information Science and Systems, 2, 3.
  - *Explores the potential of big data analytics in healthcare, focusing on its application for ethics quality improvement and decision-making processes.*
- Koh, H. C., & Tan, G. (2011). Data mining applications in healthcare. Journal of Healthcare Information Management, 19(2), 64-72.
  - *Provides insights into data mining techniques and their applications in healthcare, emphasizing their role in improving ethics quality and patient outcomes.*

**Exploring Future Trends in Bioethics Technology**


- Topol, E. J. (2012). The Creative Destruction of Medicine: How the Digital Revolution Will Create Better Health Care. Basic Books.
  - *Examines the impact of the digital revolution on healthcare, discussing future trends and the potential for technology to enhance bioethics practices.*
- Moor, J. H. (2005). Why we need better ethics for emerging technologies. Ethics and Information Technology, 7(3), 111-119.
  - *Argues for the development of robust ethical frameworks to address the challenges posed by emerging technologies in healthcare and beyond.*


***

# Review Questions

**True/False Questions:**

1. The EHR system can be customized to include specific fields for recording ethics consultations and developing standardized templates for informed consent.
True or False?

2. Training practitioners to use SOAP Notes effectively involves documenting the patient's narrative, clinical findings, ethical analysis, and planned actions.
True or False?

3. Regular audits of ethical documentation within the EHR system are not necessary for ensuring compliance with ethical standards.
True or False?

4. Data analytics can help the Bioethics Program Director identify trends in ethical issues and evaluate the impact of training programs.
True or False?

5. The director should avoid using digital tools like online platforms and video conferencing for ethics rounds and training programs.
True or False?

**Multiple-Choice Questions:**

6. Which of the following is a crucial step for integrating ethics into the EHR system for ethical documentation?
a) Ignoring customization options for the EHR
b) Collaborating with IT professionals and EHR system administrators
c) Avoiding training sessions for practitioners
d) Disregarding the development of templates for ethical documentation

7. What is a key benefit of using SOAP Notes in ethics consultations?
a) Providing vague and generalized information
b) Enhancing the quality and consistency of ethical documentation
c) Limiting the communication between practitioners
d) Ignoring the patient's narrative

**Clinical Vignettes:**

8. A patient expresses concerns about the confidentiality of their health information being recorded in the EHR system. What is the best course of action for the Bioethics Program Director?
a) Dismiss the patient's concerns as unfounded
b) Explain the measures in place to protect patient privacy and confidentiality
c) Suggest the patient avoid discussing sensitive information
d) Ignore the concerns and proceed with documentation

9. During an ethics consultation, it is discovered that the documentation of informed consent is inconsistent across different cases. What should the Bioethics Program Director do?
a) Ignore the inconsistencies and move on
b) Implement standardized templates for documenting informed consent and train practitioners on their use
c) Blame the practitioners for not following procedures
d) Discontinue the use of the EHR system for ethical documentation

10. A healthcare provider is unsure how to document an ethics consultation using SOAP Notes in the EHR system. What is the best approach for the Bioethics Program Director?
a) Tell the provider to figure it out on their own
b) Provide training and resources on how to use SOAP Notes for ethical documentation
c) Suggest the provider avoid using SOAP Notes
d) Replace SOAP Notes with a less structured method

## Correct Answers:

1. True
2. True
3. False (Regular audits of ethical documentation within the EHR system are necessary for ensuring compliance with ethical standards.)
4. True
5. False (The director should use digital tools like online platforms and video conferencing for ethics rounds and training programs.)
6. b) Collaborating with IT professionals and EHR system administrators
7. b) Enhancing the quality and consistency of ethical documentation
8. b) Explain the measures in place to protect patient privacy and confidentiality
9. b) Implement standardized templates for documenting informed consent and train practitioners on their use
10. b) Provide training and resources on how to use SOAP Notes for ethical documentation

***

# Part V: Continuous Improvement and Professional Development

## Chapter 12: Analyzing and Improving Consultation Methods

Continuous improvement in ethics consultation methods is essential to align with the Bioethics Program's mission and vision. By regularly reviewing and refining these methods, the program ensures adherence to the core bioethical principles of patient autonomy (informed consent), practitioner beneficence (maximize benefits), practitioner nonmaleficence (minimize burdens), and public justice (ensure fairness). This chapter outlines strategies for regular review and evaluation, gathering stakeholder feedback, adopting best practices, and fostering continuous education for ethics consultants. The ultimate goal is to maintain high standards in ethical decision-making, ensuring compliance with institutional policies, established medical standards of care, and legal mandates.

### Regularly Reviewing and Evaluating Processes

To ensure the effectiveness of ethics consultations, the director should implement a robust system for regular review and evaluation. This system should include:

1. **Audits**: Conduct regular audits of ethics consultations to assess the quality, consistency, and completeness of documentation. Audits can help identify discrepancies, ensure adherence to ethical standards, and provide a basis for continuous improvement.
2. **Peer Reviews**: Implement peer review processes where ethics consultants review each other's cases. Peer reviews offer a

valuable opportunity for consultants to learn from one another, share insights, and uphold a high standard of ethical practice.

3. **Feedback Surveys**: Utilize feedback surveys to gather insights from patients, families, and healthcare providers who have been involved in ethics consultations. These surveys should assess satisfaction with the consultation process, the clarity of communication, and the perceived fairness of decisions.
4. **Data Analysis:** Collect and analyze data on consultation outcomes, including resolution times, types of ethical issues addressed, and recurrence of issues. Analyzing this data helps identify trends, measure the impact of consultations, and determine areas for improvement.

## Incorporating Qualitative and Quantitative Evaluation Methods

A comprehensive evaluation approach combines both qualitative and quantitative methods:

1. **Qualitative Methods**: Conduct interviews and focus groups with stakeholders to gain deeper insights into their experiences and perceptions. These methods provide rich, detailed feedback that can uncover underlying concerns and highlight areas for enhancement.
2. **Quantitative Methods**: Use surveys and statistical analysis to obtain measurable indicators of consultation performance. Metrics such as response times, documentation completeness, and stakeholder satisfaction scores provide objective data to evaluate the effectiveness of consultation processes.

**Adapting to External Factors**:

The director should remain vigilant to external factors that may impact consultation processes:

1. **Regulatory Changes**: Stay informed about changes in healthcare regulations that may affect ethics consultation

practices. Adapting to new regulations ensures compliance and maintains the integrity of the Bioethics Program.

2. **Technological Advancements**: Embrace new technologies that can enhance consultation processes. For example, incorporating electronic health records (EHR) for documentation and using digital communication tools can improve efficiency and accessibility.
3. **Evolving Ethical Standards**: Participate in professional organizations and conferences to stay updated on evolving ethical standards. Engaging with the broader bioethics community ensures that the Bioethics Program aligns with contemporary ethical practices and thought leadership.

### Gathering Feedback and Adapting Best Practices

Feedback from stakeholders is a cornerstone of continuous improvement in ethics consultation methods. The director should establish diverse channels for collecting feedback:

1. **Anonymous Surveys**: Develop anonymous surveys for patients, families, and healthcare providers to provide candid feedback on the consultation process. Ensure that these surveys are easy to access and complete, encouraging broad participation.
2. **Interviews and Focus Groups**: Conduct interviews and focus groups with key stakeholders to explore their experiences in greater depth. These discussions can reveal nuanced perspectives that may not emerge through surveys alone.
3. **Regular Feedback Sessions**: Schedule regular feedback sessions with ethics consultants and other healthcare practitioners to discuss their experiences and suggestions. These sessions foster open communication and create a culture of collaboration and continuous improvement.

## Systematic Analysis of Feedback

Analyzing feedback requires a systematic approach:

1. **Categorize Feedback**: Organize feedback into categories such as communication, decision-making, documentation, and patient satisfaction. This categorization helps identify common themes and areas for targeted improvement.
2. **Prioritize Improvements**: Prioritize feedback based on its relevance and feasibility for implementation. Focus on changes that will have the most significant impact on consultation quality and stakeholder satisfaction.
3. **Share Feedback Summaries**: Provide feedback summaries to the ethics consultation team and other relevant stakeholders. Sharing insights fosters a collaborative approach to addressing issues and implementing improvements.

## Adapting Best Practices

Staying informed about best practices in ethics consultation is crucial:

1. **Engage with Professional Organizations**: Actively participate in professional organizations such as the American Society of Bioethics and Humanities (ASBH). These organizations provide valuable resources, training, and networking opportunities.
2. **Review Academic Literature**: Regularly review academic publications and research on ethics consultation methods. Staying informed about the latest developments helps integrate evidence-based practices into the program.
3. **Implement Best Practices**: Adapt best practices to the organization's specific context and needs. This may involve customizing protocols, training materials, and documentation templates to reflect the organization's unique environment.

## Continuous Education and Training for Ethics Consultants

Continuous education is essential for maintaining high standards in ethics consultations. The director should design comprehensive training programs that include:

1. **Workshops and Seminars**: Organize workshops and seminars that cover foundational ethical principles, case studies, and specialized topics such as end-of-life care, informed consent, and surrogate decision-making.
2. **Interactive Learning**: Utilize interactive learning methods such as simulations, role-playing exercises, and group discussions. These activities allow consultants to apply ethical principles to real-world scenarios and develop practical skills.
3. **Online Training Modules**: Develop online training modules that offer flexibility and accessibility. Modules should include video lectures, interactive quizzes, and downloadable resources. Online training enables consultants to learn at their own pace and revisit materials as needed.

## Fostering a Culture of Lifelong Learning

Promoting a culture of lifelong learning among ethics consultants is vital:

1. **Peer-to-Peer Mentoring**: Establish peer mentoring programs where experienced consultants mentor newer members. Mentoring provides guidance, support, and knowledge sharing.
2. **Journal Clubs and Discussion Groups**: Encourage consultants to participate in journal clubs and discussion groups. These forums provide opportunities to discuss recent developments in bioethics, share insights, and engage in critical thinking.
3. **Access to Resources**: Provide consultants with access to a digital library of bioethics articles, books, and case studies. Easy access to high-quality resources supports continuous learning and professional development.

## Evaluating Training Effectiveness

Regular evaluation of training programs ensures their effectiveness:

1. **Participant Feedback**: Collect feedback from training participants through surveys and interviews. Use this feedback to assess the relevance, quality, and impact of training sessions.
2. **Performance Assessments**: Conduct assessments to evaluate consultants' knowledge and skills before and after training. Assessments help measure learning outcomes and identify areas for further development.
3. **Continuous Improvement**: Use feedback and assessment results to refine training content and delivery methods. Continuous improvement ensures that training programs remain relevant and effective in addressing emerging ethical challenges.

## Ensuring Compliance and Upholding Ethical Standards

Compliance with ethical principles and legal requirements is a foundational aspect of ethics consultations. The director should ensure:

1. **Adherence to Core Bioethical Principles**: Consultations must reflect patient autonomy, practitioner beneficence, nonmaleficence, and public justice. Ethical analysis should consider these principles in every case, emphasizing informed consent, the patient's reasonable goals, and the minimization of harm.
2. **Legal and Policy Compliance**: All consultations should comply with applicable federal and state laws, as well as institutional policies. The director should regularly review and update consultation protocols to ensure they reflect current legal standards.
3. **Documentation and Transparency**: Ensure that all consultations are documented clearly and comprehensively. Documentation should capture the patient's narrative, ethical

analysis, recommendations, and decision-making process. Transparency in documentation fosters accountability and trust.

## Conclusion

Analyzing and improving ethics consultation methods is a continuous process that aligns with the Bioethics Program's mission to promote ethical decision-making in patient care. By regularly reviewing and evaluating consultation processes, gathering stakeholder feedback, adapting best practices, and providing continuous education for ethics consultants, the program can uphold the highest standards of ethical practice. These efforts ensure compliance with ethical principles, institutional policies, and legal mandates, ultimately enhancing the quality and compassion of patient care.

***

The following templates are designed to support the continuous improvement of consultation methods, gathering valuable feedback, and ensuring the ongoing professional development of ethics consultants within the Bioethics Program. By using these structured tools, the Bioethics Program Director can maintain high standards and adapt to the evolving needs of the organization.

***

## 12.1 Consultation Process Evaluation Template

**Purpose**: To systematically review and evaluate the effectiveness of ethics consultations.

**Date**: [Date]
**Prepared by**: [Name/Title]
**Department**: [Department Name]

**Consultation Overview**

- **Consultation ID**:
  [Enter unique consultation identifier.]
- **Date of Consultation**:
  [Enter the date of the ethics consultation.]
- **Consultation Participants**:
  [List the names and roles of individuals involved in the consultation.]

**Evaluation Criteria**

- **Timeliness of Response**:
  [Rate the promptness of the consultation response, e.g., 1-5 scale, with 1 being very slow and 5 being very prompt.]
- **Clarity and Thoroughness of Documentation**:
  [Rate the clarity and thoroughness of the consultation documentation, e.g., 1-5 scale.]
- **Stakeholder Satisfaction**:
  [Rate the satisfaction of involved parties, e.g., 1-5 scale.]
- **Resolution of Ethical Issues**:
  [Rate the effectiveness of the consultation in resolving ethical issues, e.g., 1-5 scale.]

**Qualitative Feedback**

- **Strengths Identified**:
  [Summarize the strengths observed in the consultation process.]

- **Areas for Improvement**:
  [Identify areas where the consultation process could be enhanced.]
- **Suggestions for Future Consultations**:
  [Provide specific suggestions for improving future consultations.]

**External Factors**

- **Regulatory Changes**:
  [Note any recent changes in healthcare regulations that may have impacted the consultation process.]
- **Technological Advancements**:
  [Describe any technological factors that may have influenced the consultation.]

**Action Plan**

- **Immediate Improvements**:
  [List any immediate actions to be taken to improve consultation processes.]
- **Long-term Strategies**:
  [Outline strategies for long-term improvements in consultation methods.]
- **Responsible Parties**:
  [Assign responsibilities for implementing the action plan.]

**Next Review Date**:
[Set a date for the next evaluation of consultation processes.]

***

## 12.2 Stakeholder Feedback Collection Form

**Purpose**: To gather structured feedback from stakeholders involved in ethics consultations.

**Date**: [Date]
**Prepared by**: [Name/Title]
**Consultation ID**: [Enter unique consultation identifier.]

**Stakeholder Information**

- **Name (Optional)**:
  [Enter stakeholder's name or leave blank for anonymous feedback.]
- **Role in Consultation**:
  [Describe the stakeholder's role, e.g., patient, family member, healthcare provider.]

**Feedback Questions**

- **Overall Satisfaction**:
  [Rate your overall satisfaction with the consultation process, e.g., 1-5 scale.]
- **Effectiveness of Communication**:
  [Rate the effectiveness of communication during the consultation, e.g., 1-5 scale.]
- **Clarity of Ethical Recommendations**:
  [Rate how clearly the ethical recommendations were communicated, e.g., 1-5 scale.]
- **Outcome Satisfaction**:
  [Rate your satisfaction with the outcome of the consultation, e.g., 1-5 scale.]

**Open-Ended Feedback**

- What aspects of the consultation were most helpful?
  [Provide an open-ended response.]
- Were there any challenges or issues that were not addressed?
  [Provide an open-ended response.]
- How could the consultation process be improved?
  [Provide an open-ended response.]

**Additional Comments**

- Please share any additional thoughts or suggestions.
  [Provide an open-ended response.]

***

## 12.3 Continuous Education and Training Plan

**Purpose**: To outline the plan for continuous education and training of ethics consultants.

**Date**: [Date]
**Prepared by**: [Name/Title]
**Department**: [Department Name]

**Training Objectives**

- **Core Competencies**:
  [List the key competencies that the training program aims to develop or enhance.]
- **Specific Topics Covered**:
  [Identify the topics to be covered, e.g., foundational ethical principles, end-of-life care.]

**Training Methods**

- **Workshops and Seminars**:
  [Describe planned in-person workshops and seminars.]
- **Online Courses and Modules**:
  [List available online training modules and courses.]
- **Interactive Activities**:
  [Describe planned activities such as role-playing, case studies, and simulations.]

**Training Schedule**

- **Monthly/Quarterly Training Sessions**:
  [Provide the schedule for regular training sessions.]
- **Special Training Events**:
  [List any special events or guest lectures planned.]

**Resources and Materials**

- **Training Materials Provided**:
  [List materials to be provided, e.g., handouts, online resources, case study collections.]
- **Access to Online Resources**:
  [Describe how consultants can access digital libraries, e-learning courses, etc.]

**Evaluation and Feedback**

- **Participant Feedback**:
  [Describe how participant feedback will be collected and used.]
- **Performance Assessments**:
  [Outline methods for assessing the effectiveness of the training.]

**Continuous Learning Opportunities**

- **Informal Learning Activities**:
  [List opportunities for informal learning, e.g., peer mentoring, discussion groups.]
- **Encouraging Lifelong Learning**:
  [Describe how a culture of lifelong learning will be promoted.]

**Review and Update Schedule**

- **Next Training Plan Review**:
  [Set a date for reviewing and updating the training plan.]

***

## Further Readings and References


### Regularly Reviewing and Evaluating Processes

- Deming, W. E. (1986). Out of the Crisis. MIT Press.
  - *Introduces Deming's principles of quality management and continuous improvement, emphasizing the importance of regular review and evaluation of processes to enhance performance.*
- Langley, G. J., Moen, R. D., Nolan, K. M., Nolan, T. W., Norman, C. L., & Provost, L. P. (2009). The Improvement Guide: A Practical Approach to Enhancing Organizational Performance (2nd ed.). Jossey-Bass.
  - *Provides a practical approach to improving organizational performance through systematic process evaluation and iterative improvements.*

### Gathering Feedback and Adapting Best Practices

- Batalden, P. B., & Davidoff, F. (2007). What is "quality improvement" and how can it transform healthcare? Quality and Safety in Health Care, 16(1), 2-3.
  - *Discusses the concept of quality improvement in healthcare and its transformative potential, highlighting the importance of gathering feedback and adapting best practices.*
- Donabedian, A. (2003). An Introduction to Quality Assurance in Health Care. Oxford University Press.
  - *Explores the principles of quality assurance in healthcare, emphasizing the role of feedback in refining and adopting best practices for better outcomes.*

### Continuous Education and Training for Ethics Consultants

- Frenk, J., Chen, L., Bhutta, Z. A., Cohen, J., Crisp, N., Evans, T., ... & Zurayk, H. (2010). Health professionals for a new century: transforming education to strengthen health systems in an interdependent world. The Lancet, 376(9756), 1923-1958.
  - *Advocates for transforming health professional education to meet the needs of modern health systems, stressing the importance of continuous learning for ethics consultants.*
- Steinert, Y. (Ed.). (2014). Faculty Development in the Health Professions: A Focus on Research and Practice. Springer.
  - *Focuses on faculty development in health professions, providing insights into effective training and continuous education for ethics consultants.*

***

# Chapter 13: Personal and Professional Growth

Personal and professional growth are critical for leaders in bioethics, as they navigate the evolving landscape of healthcare ethics. This chapter explores the strategies for staying informed on regulatory standards and ethical norms, participating in professional conferences and continuing education, and balancing professional responsibilities with personal well-being. By focusing on these areas, the director of a Bioethics Program can ensure alignment with the mission and vision of the organization, uphold the four core bioethical principles, and foster a culture of ethical awareness and continuous improvement.

## Staying Informed on Regulatory Standards and Ethical Norms

To stay abreast of regulatory standards and ethical norms, the director should implement a structured approach to knowledge management:

1. **Regular Review of Laws and Guidelines**: Establish a routine for reviewing relevant laws, regulations, and guidelines. This can include updates from regulatory bodies, healthcare standards organizations, and ethical guidelines from professional associations.

2. **Internal Knowledge Base**: Develop an internal knowledge management system that houses essential resources, such as policy documents, regulatory updates, and best practice guidelines. This centralized repository should be easily accessible to all team members, ensuring that everyone has up-to-date information at their fingertips.

3. **Subscription to Professional Journals and Newsletters**: Subscribe to relevant journals, newsletters, and online platforms

that provide regular updates on bioethics, healthcare regulations, and legal developments. Curate and disseminate this information to the team, fostering an informed and engaged workforce.

4. **Engagement with Professional Organizations**: Actively participate in organizations such as the Association of Bioethics Program Directors (ABPD) and the American Society of Bioethics and Humanities (ASBH). These organizations offer valuable resources, networking opportunities, and insights into emerging trends and challenges in bioethics.

### Promoting a Culture of Continuous Learning and Improvement:

Creating a culture that values continuous learning and improvement is vital for staying aligned with current ethical standards:

1. **Regular Training Sessions:** Organize training sessions and workshops that focus on the latest regulatory changes and ethical guidelines. These sessions should be interactive and provide opportunities for discussion and clarification.
2. **Encouraging Experimentation and Innovation**: Foster an environment where practitioners feel empowered to explore new ideas, experiment with innovative approaches, and implement best practices. Recognize and celebrate innovative behavior that enhances the Bioethics Program.
3. **Continuous Feedback Mechanisms**: Implement continuous feedback mechanisms to capture insights from team members about regulatory changes and ethical challenges. Encourage open dialogue and collaboration to address these challenges effectively.

### Tracking and Disseminating Updates

1. **Tracking Regulatory Changes**: Assign responsibility for monitoring regulatory changes to a designated team member or committee. This ensures that updates are tracked systematically and communicated promptly.

2. **Regular Updates**: Provide regular updates to the team through meetings, emails, and internal bulletins. Make use of digital platforms to disseminate information efficiently and ensure that all team members are aware of the latest developments.
3. **Workshops on New Standards**: Conduct workshops to discuss the implications of new regulations and guidelines. These workshops should focus on practical applications and strategies for integrating new standards into existing practices.

## Participating in Professional Conferences and Continuing Education

Participation in professional conferences and continuing education is crucial for personal and professional development:

1. **Knowledge Sharing**: Conferences provide a platform for sharing knowledge, insights, and experiences with peers. Presenting at conferences enhances the visibility of the Bioethics Program and establishes the director as a thought leader in the field.
2. **Networking Opportunities**: Engaging with other professionals at conferences allows for networking and building relationships. These connections can lead to collaborative projects, research opportunities, and the sharing of best practices.
3. **Staying Informed**: Attending sessions and workshops at conferences helps the director stay informed about the latest developments, research, and innovations in bioethics. This knowledge is essential for ensuring that the Bioethics Program remains relevant and effective.

## Developing a Strategic Plan for Conference Engagement

To maximize the benefits of conference participation, the director should develop a strategic plan:

1. **Identify Key Conferences**: Identify key conferences that align with the goals and interests of the Bioethics Program. Prioritize

events that offer opportunities for learning, networking, and collaboration.

2. **Set Participation Goals**: Set clear goals for participation, such as presenting a paper, attending specific sessions, or meeting potential collaborators. Having defined objectives ensures that conference attendance is purposeful and impactful.
3. **Follow-up Plan**: Create a follow-up plan to implement and share the knowledge gained at conferences. This can involve debriefing sessions with the team, sharing resources and insights, and incorporating new ideas into the program's practices.

### Encouraging Team Participation

1. **Supporting Attendance**: Encourage and support team members to attend professional conferences. Provide financial support, facilitate time off for professional development, and recognize the importance of continuous learning.
2. **Sharing Knowledge**: Encourage team members who attend conferences to share their learnings with the rest of the team. Organize presentations or informal discussions where attendees can discuss what they learned and how it can be applied to the Bioethics Program.
3. **Continuing Education Credits**: Promote opportunities for earning continuing education credits through conference participation. These credits contribute to professional development and maintain certification for ethics consultants.

## Balancing Professional Responsibilities with Personal Well-being

**Prioritizing Self-care and Work-life Balance**:

The well-being of the director is crucial for sustainable and effective leadership:

1. **Time Management:** Develop effective time management strategies to balance professional responsibilities with personal

life. Prioritize tasks, set realistic deadlines, and avoid overcommitting.

2. **Delegation**: Delegate tasks to team members to prevent burnout and ensure a balanced workload. Trusting the team with responsibilities empowers them and fosters a collaborative work environment.
3. **Setting Boundaries**: Establish clear boundaries between work and personal life. Allocate time for relaxation, hobbies, and activities that promote well-being. Ensure that work commitments do not encroach on personal time.

**Promoting a Culture of Self-care:**

1. **Awareness Campaigns**: Launch awareness campaigns that highlight the importance of self-care and work-life balance. Encourage team members to take breaks, manage stress, and prioritize their health.
2. **Training and Support**: Provide training on stress management, mindfulness, and resilience. Offer resources and support for team members to manage their well-being effectively.
3. **Recognition of Healthy Behavior**: Recognize and celebrate team members who demonstrate a commitment to self-care. Positive reinforcement encourages a culture where well-being is valued.

## Implementing Organizational Policies for Work-life Balance

1. **Flexible Working Hours**: Introduce flexible working hours to accommodate the personal needs of team members. Flexibility in scheduling can reduce stress and enhance job satisfaction.
2. **Remote Work Options:** Offer remote work options where feasible. Remote work provides flexibility and can help team members balance professional and personal commitments.

3. **Sufficient Vacation Time**: Ensure that team members have access to sufficient vacation time. Encourage them to take time off to recharge and disconnect from work.

## Leading by Example

1. **Demonstrating Self-care**: Lead by example by prioritizing self-care and maintaining a healthy work-life balance. The director's actions set the tone for the rest of the team.
2. **Checking in with Team Members**: Regularly check in with team members about their well-being. Provide support, resources, and a listening ear to those who may be struggling with stress or burnout.
3. **Creating a Supportive Environment**: Foster a supportive work environment where team members feel comfortable discussing their well-being. Encourage open communication and provide resources for managing stress and maintaining health.

## Conclusion

Personal and professional growth are essential for the success of the Bioethics Program and its alignment with the mission and vision statements. By staying informed on regulatory standards and ethical norms, participating in professional conferences and continuing education, and balancing professional responsibilities with personal well-being, the director can lead the Bioethics Program effectively. These strategies ensure that ethical considerations are integrated into patient care and decision-making, promoting a culture of ethical awareness, continuous learning, and high-quality, compassionate patient care.

***

The following templates support the personal and professional growth of the Bioethics Program Director and their team, helping them stay informed, engage in continuous learning, and maintain a healthy work-life balance. By using these structured tools, the director can foster a culture of continuous improvement and well-being within the Bioethics Program.

***

## 13.1 Regulatory Standards and Ethical Norms Tracking Template

**Purpose**: To systematically track updates on regulatory standards and ethical norms and ensure that the Bioethics Program stays informed and compliant.

**Date**: [Date]
**Prepared by**: [Name/Title]
**Department**: [Department Name]

**Regulatory Update Information**

- **Source of Update**:
  [Identify the source, e.g., government agency, professional organization, journal.]
- **Title of Regulation/Guideline**:
  [Enter the name of the regulation or guideline.]
- **Date of Publication/Update**:
  [Enter the date when the regulation or guideline was published or updated.]
- **Summary of Changes/Updates**:
  [Provide a brief summary of the changes or updates.]

**Impact on Bioethics Program**

- **Relevant Areas of Impact**:
  [Identify the specific areas of the Bioethics Program affected by the update.]
- **Required Actions**:
  [List any actions that need to be taken to comply with the update.]
- **Responsible Parties**:
  [Assign responsibilities for implementing the required actions.]

**Dissemination and Communication**

- **Team Members Informed**:
  [List the team members who need to be informed about the update.]
- **Communication Method**:
  [Describe how the information will be communicated, e.g., email, meeting, newsletter.]
- **Follow-Up**:
  [Set a date for follow-up to ensure that the necessary actions have been taken.]

**Review and Integration**

- **Policy/Procedure Adjustments**:
  [Note any adjustments needed in existing policies or procedures.]
- **Training Requirements**:
  [Identify any training needed to ensure compliance with the update.]
- **Next Review Date**:
  [Set a date for the next review of this regulation or guideline.]

***

## 13.2 Professional Development and Continuing Education Plan

---

**Purpose**: To outline and track participation in professional development and continuing education activities.

**Date**: [Date]
**Prepared by**: [Name/Title]
**Department**: [Department Name]

**Professional Development Goals**

- **Short-Term Goals**:
  [List specific goals for professional development over the next year.]
- **Long-Term Goals**:
  [List broader professional development goals for the next 3-5 years.]

**Continuing Education Activities**

- **Conferences and Workshops**:
  [List planned conferences and workshops, including dates and locations.]
- **Online Courses and Webinars**:
  [List any online courses or webinars to be completed.]
- **Professional Organization Memberships**:
  [List memberships in professional organizations and any relevant activities.]

**Budget and Resources**

- **Budget Allocation**:
  [Outline the budget for professional development activities.]
- **Support Resources**:
  [List any resources available to support professional development, such as time off, funding, etc.]

**Participation and Reflection**

- **Activities Completed**:
  [Track completed activities, including dates and key takeaways.]
- **Impact on Professional Growth**:
  [Reflect on how each activity has contributed to personal and professional growth.]
- **Application to Bioethics Program**:
  [Note how the knowledge and skills gained can be applied to improve the Bioethics Program.]

**Next Steps**

- **Further Learning Opportunities**:
  [Identify additional learning opportunities to pursue.]
- **Sharing Knowledge with Team**:
  [Plan how to share insights and knowledge with the team.]
- **Review and Update**:
  [Set a date for the next review and update of the professional development plan.]

***

## 13.3 Work-Life Balance Assessment Template

**Purpose**: To assess and plan for balancing professional responsibilities with personal well-being.

**Date**: [Date]
**Prepared by**: [Name/Title]
**Department**: [Department Name]

**Current Workload and Responsibilities**

- **Key Responsibilities**:
  [List current professional responsibilities.]
- **Time Allocation**:
  [Estimate the amount of time spent on each responsibility per week.]

**Personal Well-Being Assessment**

- **Stress Levels**:
  [Rate current stress levels on a scale of 1-10.]
- **Physical Health**:
  [Note any physical health concerns related to work.]
- **Mental Health**:
  [Note any mental health concerns related to work.]

**Strategies for Improvement**

- **Time Management Techniques**:
  [List time management techniques to implement, e.g., prioritization, scheduling.]
- **Delegation Opportunities**:
  [Identify tasks that can be delegated to others.]
- **Setting Boundaries**:
  [Describe any boundaries that need to be set, such as work hours, availability, etc.]

**Self-Care and Personal Well-Being**

- **Self-Care Practices**:
  [List current self-care practices and any new practices to implement.]
- **Work-Life Balance Goals**:
  [Set specific goals for improving work-life balance.]

**Review and Adjustment**

- **Progress Check**:
  [Set a date for reviewing progress on work-life balance.]
- **Adjustments Needed**:
  [Note any adjustments needed to better balance work and personal life.]

***

## Further Readings and References

### Staying Informed on Regulatory Standards and Ethical Norms


- Jonsen, A. R. (2003). The Birth of Bioethics. Oxford University Press.
  - *Chronicles the development of bioethics as a field, emphasizing the importance of staying informed about regulatory standards and ethical norms.*
- Grinnell, F. (1992). The Scientific Attitude. Guilford Press.
  - *Explores the scientific attitude and its relevance to ethical practice, highlighting the need for continuous learning and adherence to ethical norms.*


### Participating in Professional Conferences and Continuing Education


- Bligh, J., & Parsell, G. (1999). Multiprofessional working: learning from experience. Medical Education, 33(9), 716-723.
  - *Discusses the benefits of multiprofessional learning and collaboration, encouraging participation in professional conferences and continuing education.*
- Knowles, M. S., Holton, E. F., & Swanson, R. A. (2011). The Adult Learner: The Definitive Classic in Adult Education and Human Resource Development (7th ed.). Butterworth-Heinemann.
  - *A seminal text on adult learning principles, offering insights into effective continuing education for professionals.*


### Balancing Professional Responsibilities with Personal Well-being


- Goleman, D. (1995). Emotional Intelligence: Why It Can Matter More Than IQ. Bantam Books.
  - *Highlights the importance of emotional intelligence in balancing professional responsibilities and personal well-being.*

- Maslach, C., & Leiter, M. P. (2016). The Truth About Burnout: How Organizations Cause Personal Stress and What to Do About It. Jossey-Bass.
  - *Examines the causes of burnout and offers strategies for managing stress and maintaining personal well-being in professional settings.*

***

# Chapter 14: Leading with Integrity and Compassion

Leading with integrity and compassion is fundamental to the success of the Bioethics Program and is essential for fostering a culture of ethical awareness and responsibility. This chapter will explore the principles and practices of ethical leadership, strategies for building trust and credibility, and the importance of leading by example and inspiring others. By focusing on these aspects, the director can ensure that ethical considerations are at the forefront of every decision and action, enhancing the quality and impact of the Bioethics Program.

## Ethical Leadership in Healthcare

Ethical leadership in healthcare is the practice of guiding the Bioethics Program with a commitment to the four core bioethical principles: patient autonomy (informed consent), practitioner beneficence (maximize benefits), practitioner nonmaleficence (minimize burdens), and public justice (ensure fairness). The director must demonstrate integrity, transparency, and accountability in their actions and decisions:

1. **Integrity**: Leading with integrity involves consistently aligning actions with ethical standards, regardless of external pressures or challenges. The director should be a role model for ethical behavior, upholding the values of honesty, fairness, and respect in all interactions.

2. **Transparency**: Ethical leadership requires openness in decision-making processes. The director should ensure that decisions are made transparently, with clear communication of the rationale and factors considered. This approach helps to build trust and accountability.

3. **Accountability**: The director must be accountable for their actions and the actions of the Bioethics Program. This includes taking responsibility for mistakes, learning from them, and implementing changes to prevent future errors.

## Promoting Ethical Leadership Within the Organization

1. **Training and Support**: Provide regular training on ethical leadership principles for all staff members. This training should include scenarios and role-playing exercises that challenge participants to make ethical decisions in complex situations.
2. **Ethical Reflection**: Encourage self-reflection and peer feedback as a means of promoting ethical awareness. The director should create opportunities for team members to discuss ethical challenges they face and explore solutions collaboratively.
3. **Recognition and Celebration**: Acknowledge and celebrate ethical behavior within the organization. Recognizing individuals who demonstrate strong ethical leadership reinforces the importance of these values and encourages others to follow suit.

## Ongoing Self-reflection and Personal Growth

1. **Regular Self-assessment**: The director should engage in regular self-assessment to evaluate their adherence to ethical principles. Seeking feedback from peers and mentors can provide valuable insights into areas for improvement.
2. **Commitment to Learning:** Ethical leadership is a dynamic process that requires continuous learning. The director should stay informed about emerging ethical issues, new research, and best practices in bioethics. Engaging in professional development opportunities and attending conferences can enhance the director's knowledge and skills.
3. **Alignment with Ethical Principles**: The director should continually strive to align their actions and decisions with the core bioethical principles. This alignment ensures that the

Bioethics Program consistently promotes patient autonomy, beneficence, nonmaleficence, and justice.

## Advocating for Ethical Practices

1. **Integrating Ethics into Organizational Strategy**: The director should work to embed ethical considerations into the strategic planning and policy development of the organization. By advocating for ethical practices at all levels, the director can ensure that the organization's mission and vision are consistently reflected in its operations.
2. **Ethics Committees and Consultation**: The director should support the establishment and maintenance of ethics committees and consultation services. These committees play a critical role in addressing ethical dilemmas and providing guidance to healthcare practitioners.
3. **Ethical Decision-making Frameworks**: Implementing ethical decision-making frameworks can guide practitioners in making ethically sound decisions. These frameworks should be incorporated into training programs and used regularly in ethics consultations.

## Building Trust and Credibility

Trust is the foundation of effective leadership and successful collaboration within the Bioethics Program:

1. **Consistency and Reliability**: Trust is built through consistent and reliable actions. The director should be dependable, follow through on commitments, and demonstrate consistency in ethical behavior.
2. **Open Communication**: Transparent and honest communication is key to building trust. The director should ensure that information is shared openly with stakeholders, and that the rationale behind decisions is clearly explained.
3. **Active Listening**: Building trust also involves actively listening to the concerns and perspectives of others. The director should

create a safe environment for stakeholders to express their views and respond with empathy and support.

### Promoting a Culture of Trust and Credibility

1. **Awareness Campaigns**: Develop awareness campaigns that highlight the importance of trust and credibility within the Bioethics Program. Use case studies and real-life examples to illustrate how trust and transparency lead to better ethical outcomes.
2. **Regular Feedback**: Encourage regular feedback from stakeholders about the Bioethics Program and its leadership. Use this feedback to make improvements and demonstrate a commitment to accountability.
3. **Recognition of Ethical Behavior**: Acknowledge and reward individuals who consistently demonstrate ethical behavior and contribute to building trust within the organization. Recognition can take the form of awards, public acknowledgments, or professional development opportunities.

### Transparency in Decision-Making

1. **Clear Decision-making Processes**: Establish clear and consistent processes for decision-making within the Bioethics Program. Ensure that these processes are well-documented and communicated to all stakeholders.
2. **Inclusive Decision-making**: Involve relevant stakeholders in the decision-making process. This inclusion fosters a sense of ownership and respect, enhancing trust and collaboration.
3. **Documentation and Reporting**: Maintain thorough documentation of decisions and the reasoning behind them. Regular reporting to stakeholders about decisions and outcomes promotes transparency and accountability.

### Leading by Example and Inspiring Others

1. **Setting High Standards:** The director should set high standards for ethical behavior and hold themselves and others accountable

to these standards. This includes adhering to the principles of honesty, integrity, and respect in all interactions.

2. **Demonstrating Empathy and Compassion**: Ethical leadership is rooted in empathy and compassion. The director should demonstrate these qualities in their interactions with patients, families, and colleagues, showing understanding and concern for their needs and well-being.
3. **Accountability for Actions**: Leading by example means taking responsibility for one's actions. The director should be willing to admit mistakes, learn from them, and make the necessary corrections.

## Inspiring a Shared Vision

1. **Articulating a Compelling Vision**: The director should communicate a clear and compelling vision for the Bioethics Program, emphasizing the importance of ethical practices in achieving the organization's mission. This vision should inspire and motivate stakeholders to commit to ethical excellence.
2. **Engaging Stakeholders**: Involve stakeholders in shaping the vision and goals of the Bioethics Program. Engagement fosters a sense of ownership and alignment with the program's objectives.
3. **Regular Communication**: Consistently communicate the vision and goals of the Bioethics Program to stakeholders. Use various platforms, such as meetings, newsletters, and presentations, to reinforce the importance of ethical practices.

## Recognizing and Celebrating Contributions

1. **Acknowledging Achievements**: Recognize and celebrate the achievements of team members and stakeholders who demonstrate ethical behavior. Public acknowledgment and appreciation reinforce the value of ethical practices.
2. **Creating Opportunities for Growth**: Provide opportunities for professional development and growth for individuals who

contribute to the Bioethics Program. This investment in their development encourages ongoing commitment to ethical principles.

3. **Building a Supportive Environment**: Foster a supportive environment where team members feel valued and respected. Encouragement and positive reinforcement create a culture where ethical behavior is the norm.

**Conclusion**

Leading with integrity and compassion is essential for the success of the Bioethics Program. By modeling ethical behavior, building trust and credibility, and inspiring others, the director can create a culture of ethical awareness and responsibility. These efforts ensure that the Bioethics Program aligns with its mission and vision, promoting patient autonomy (informed consent), practitioner beneficence (maximize benefits), practitioner nonmaleficence (minimize burdens), and public justice (ensure fairness). Ethical leadership enhances the quality of patient care, supports the well-being of healthcare professionals, and contributes to the overall effectiveness of the healthcare organization.

***

The following forms and templates are designed to support the director in leading with integrity and compassion, building trust, and inspiring others within the Bioethics Program. By using these tools regularly, the director can ensure they are consistently practicing and promoting cthical leadership throughout the organization.

***

## 14.1 Stakeholder Trust-Building Checklist

**Purpose**: To ensure that the director is consistently taking actions to build and maintain trust with stakeholders.

**Date**: [Date]
**Name**: [Director's Name]
**Department**: [Department Name]

**Communication**

1. Am I communicating openly and honestly with stakeholders?
   ☐ Yes
   ☐ No
   [Comments/Examples]
2. Do I regularly update stakeholders on important decisions and developments?
   ☐ Yes
   ☐ No
   [Comments/Examples]
3. Am I transparent about the decision-making process and outcomes?
   ☐ Yes
   ☐ No
   [Comments/Examples]

**Reliability**

4. Do I consistently deliver on my commitments and promises?
   ☐ Yes
   ☐ No
   [Comments/Examples]

5. Am I dependable and available when stakeholders need support or guidance?
   ☐ Yes
   ☐ No
   [Comments/Examples]

**Empathy and Support**

6. Do I actively listen to the concerns and perspectives of stakeholders?
   ☐ Yes
   ☐ No
   [Comments/Examples]
7. Do I respond to stakeholder concerns with empathy and support?
   ☐ Yes
   ☐ No
   [Comments/Examples]
8. Am I proactive in addressing issues that could affect trust and credibility?
   ☐ Yes
   ☐ No
   [Comments/Examples]

**Recognition and Validation**

9. Do I recognize and validate the contributions and efforts of stakeholders?
   ☐ Yes
   ☐ No
   [Comments/Examples]
10. Am I fostering an environment where stakeholders feel valued and respected?
    ☐ Yes
    ☐ No
    [Comments/Examples]

**Continuous Improvement**

11. Am I seeking feedback from stakeholders to improve trust and collaboration?
    - ☐ Yes
    - ☐ No

    [Comments/Examples]

12. Do I make adjustments based on feedback to strengthen relationships with stakeholders?
    - ☐ Yes
    - ☐ No

    [Comments/Examples]

**Next Review Date**

- Set a date for the next trust-building checklist review.
  [Date]

***

## 14.2 Recognition and Inspiration Log

**Purpose**: To track efforts to recognize team members and inspire ethical practices within the Bioethics Program.

**Date**: [Date]
**Name**: [Director's Name]
**Department**: [Department Name]

**Recognition Efforts**

- Team Member/Stakeholder Recognized:
  [Name]
- **Reason for Recognition**:
  [Describe the ethical behavior or contribution recognized]
- **Method of Recognition**:
  [How was recognition given? E.g., public acknowledgment, written note, award]
- Date of Recognition:
  [Date]

**Inspiration Initiatives**

- **Initiative**:
  [Describe the initiative to inspire ethical behavior, e.g., a speech, a workshop, an event]
- **Audience**:
  [Who was inspired? E.g., team members, stakeholders]
- **Outcome/Impact**:
  [Describe the impact or response]
- **Follow-Up Actions**:
  [Any follow-up actions needed?]

**Reflection and Next Steps**

- **What went well?**
  [Reflect on what was successful]

- **What could be improved?**
  [Identify areas for improvement]
- **Next Steps for Recognition/Inspiration**:
  [Outline the next actions for continuing recognition and inspiration]

**Next Log Review Date**

- Set a date for reviewing the log and planning future recognition and inspiration efforts.
  [Date]

***

## Further Readings and References


### Ethical Leadership in Healthcare

- Shapiro, J. P., & Gross, S. J. (2013). Ethical Educational Leadership in Turbulent Times: (Re)Solving Moral Dilemmas (2nd ed.). Lawrence Erlbaum Associates.
  - *Addresses the challenges of ethical leadership in turbulent times, offering solutions to moral dilemmas in healthcare education.*
- Gallagher, A., & Hodge, S. (Eds.). (2012). Ethics, Law and Professional Issues: A Practice-Based Approach for Health Professionals. Palgrave Macmillan.
  - *Provides a practice-based approach to ethics, law, and professional issues, emphasizing the importance of ethical leadership in healthcare.*

### Building Trust and Credibility

- Covey, S. R., & Merrill, R. R. (2006). The Speed of Trust: The One Thing That Changes Everything. Free Press.
  - *Explores the concept of trust and its impact on organizational success, highlighting strategies for building trust and credibility in leadership.*
- Mayer, R. C., Davis, J. H., & Schoorman, F. D. (1995). An integrative model of organizational trust. Academy of Management Review, 20(3), 709-734.
  - *Presents an integrative model of organizational trust, offering insights into the factors that build and sustain trust within organizations.*

### Leading by Example and Inspiring Others


- Kouzes, J. M., & Posner, B. Z. (2017). The Leadership Challenge: How to Make Extraordinary Things Happen in Organizations (6th ed.). Wiley.
  - *Provides a comprehensive guide to leadership, emphasizing the importance of leading by example and inspiring others to achieve extraordinary results.*
- Burns, J. M. (1978). Leadership. Harper & Row.
  - *A seminal work on leadership that explores the transformative power of leadership and its role in inspiring and motivating others.*


***

# Review Questions

**True/False Questions:**

1. Regular review and evaluation of consultation processes are essential for continuous improvement in ethics consultations.
True or False?

2. Gathering feedback from patients, families, and healthcare providers is not necessary for improving ethics consultation methods.
True or False?

3. Continuous education and training help ethics consultants remain knowledgeable and prepared to address complex ethical dilemmas.
True or False?

4. The director should not consider external factors such as changes in healthcare regulations when reviewing consultation processes.
True or False?

5. Combining qualitative and quantitative evaluation methods provides a comprehensive assessment of consultation effectiveness.
True or False?

**Multiple-Choice Questions:**

6. Which of the following is a crucial component of a comprehensive review system for ethics consultations?
a) Ignoring feedback from stakeholders
b) Establishing a set of metrics and benchmarks for evaluating performance
c) Disregarding the timeliness of responses
d) Avoiding the use of statistical analysis

7. What is an effective method for ensuring continuous education and training for ethics consultants?
a) Providing only one-time training sessions
b) Using a variety of methods such as workshops, seminars, and online courses
c) Limiting training to theoretical knowledge only
d) Ignoring the specific needs and interests of the audience

**Clinical Vignettes:**

8. A patient expresses dissatisfaction with the outcome of an ethics consultation, feeling their perspective was not adequately considered. What is the best course of action for the Bioethics Program Director?
a) Ignore the patient's concerns
b) Gather feedback from the patient and involved parties to understand the issue and identify areas for improvement
c) Blame the ethics consultant for the dissatisfaction
d) Discontinue the feedback collection process

9. During a review of consultation processes, it is found that documentation is often incomplete and lacks clarity. What should the Bioethics Program Director do?
a) Ignore the documentation issues
b) Develop standardized templates and provide training on thorough documentation
c) Blame the practitioners for not completing documentation
d) Avoid making any changes to the documentation process

10. A new ethics consultant is struggling with the complexity of cases and feels unprepared. What is the best approach for the Bioethics Program Director?
a) Suggest the consultant handle fewer cases
b) Provide additional training, mentoring, and access to resources
c) Ignore the consultant's concerns
d) Reassign the consultant to administrative tasks only

## Correct Answers:

1. True
2. False (Gathering feedback from patients, families, and healthcare providers is necessary for improving ethics consultation methods.)
3. True
4. False (The director should consider external factors such as changes in healthcare regulations when reviewing consultation processes.)
5. True
6. b) Establishing a set of metrics and benchmarks for evaluating performance
7. b) Using a variety of methods such as workshops, seminars, and online courses
8. b) Gather feedback from the patient and involved parties to understand the issue and identify areas for improvement
9. b) Develop standardized templates and provide training on thorough documentation
10. b) Provide additional training, mentoring, and access to resources

***

# Part VI: Practical Tools and Resources

## Chapter 15: Practical Tools for Bioethics Program Directors

Practical tools and resources are essential for Bioethics Program Directors to develop, implement, and sustain policies and procedures that align with the program's mission and vision. This chapter provides comprehensive guidance on utilizing templates, checklists, and other resources to enhance policy development, ensure effective documentation, and support ethics education and training. By leveraging these tools, the director can promote the core bioethical principles of patient autonomy (informed consent), practitioner beneficence (maximize benefits), practitioner nonmaleficence (minimize burdens), and public justice (ensure fairness), ensuring compliance with medical standards of care, institutional policies, and legal mandates.

### Templates and Checklists for Policy Development

Developing and implementing effective policies is critical to the Bioethics Program's success. Policies provide a framework that guides decision-making and ensures consistent application of ethical standards. Templates and checklists offer a structured approach, making it easier to create comprehensive, clear, and consistent policies:

1. **Purpose and Scope**: Templates should include sections that clearly define the policy's objectives and the scope of its application. This clarity helps ensure that the policy addresses the relevant ethical issues and is applied consistently across the organization.

2. **Definitions**: Key terms should be defined to ensure that all stakeholders understand the policy's language and intent. This is crucial for avoiding misunderstandings and ensuring that the policy is interpreted and implemented correctly.
3. **Procedures and Responsibilities**: A well-structured policy should outline the specific procedures to be followed and clearly assign responsibilities. This delineation of roles ensures accountability and facilitates the effective implementation of the policy.
4. **Compliance and Review**: Policies should include mechanisms for regular review and compliance monitoring. Checklists can help track adherence to the policy and identify areas for improvement, ensuring the policy remains relevant and effective.

## Enhancing Quality and Consistency

Using templates and checklists ensures that all necessary components are included in policy documents, which helps maintain high standards and alignment with organizational and ethical guidelines:

1. **Standardization**: Templates create a standardized format for policies, making them easier to read, understand, and implement. Standardization promotes consistency, which is essential for training, compliance, and communication.
2. **Thoroughness**: Checklists ensure that all relevant aspects are considered during policy development. This thorough approach minimizes the risk of overlooking critical elements, such as compliance with legal standards, ethical principles, and practical considerations.
3. **Training and Familiarity**: When practitioners are familiar with a standardized policy format, training becomes more straightforward, and compliance increases. Consistent use of templates helps embed the organization's values and standards in everyday practice.

**Promoting the Use of Templates and Checklists**:

To maximize their benefits, the director should actively promote the use of templates and checklists across the organization:

1. **Awareness Campaigns**: Develop campaigns that highlight the importance and benefits of structured policy development. Use real-life examples to show how templates and checklists have enhanced policy quality and compliance.
2. **Training and Support**: Provide regular training on using these tools effectively. Offer workshops, seminars, and hands-on sessions to demonstrate how templates and checklists can be utilized in policy development.
3. **Recognition**: Recognize and reward staff members who demonstrate effective use of these tools. Acknowledgment of good practice encourages others to adopt these methods and contributes to a culture of excellence.

## SOAP Notes and Documentation Guidelines

SOAP (Subjective, Objective, Assessment, Plan) Notes provide a standardized format for documenting ethics consultations. They are essential for ensuring that all relevant information is captured and that the consultation process is transparent, accountable, and aligned with ethical standards:

**(S) Subjective**: This section captures the patient's narrative, including their understanding of their condition, treatment options, and concerns. It reflects the principle of patient autonomy by ensuring the patient's voice is heard and considered in decision-making.

**(O) Objective**: Documenting clinical findings and observations provides an accurate and unbiased account of the patient's condition. This objectivity is crucial for maintaining credibility and supporting the principles of beneficence and nonmaleficence.

**(A) Assessment**: The ethical analysis section assesses the ethical issues involved, considering patient autonomy, beneficence, nonmaleficence, and justice. This analysis guides the development of recommendations and supports ethical decision-making.

**(P) Plan**: Outlining the planned actions and follow-up ensures that ethical recommendations are implemented and monitored. This planning is essential for addressing ethical issues effectively and ensuring accountability.

## Importance of Comprehensive Documentation

Thorough documentation is vital for communication and decision-making in ethics consultations:

1. **Transparency**: Comprehensive SOAP Notes provide a clear record of the consultation, making the decision-making process transparent. This transparency helps build trust with patients, families, and healthcare providers.
2. **Accountability**: Accurate documentation holds all parties accountable for their actions and decisions. It provides a record that can be reviewed and evaluated, ensuring that ethical standards are upheld.
3. **Communication**: SOAP Notes facilitate communication among the healthcare team, ensuring that everyone is informed about the patient's situation, the ethical issues, and the recommended actions.

## Training and Support for Effective Documentation

The director should provide training and support to ensure that practitioners use SOAP Notes effectively:

1. **Practical Exercises**: Incorporate practical exercises and role-playing scenarios in training sessions. These activities allow practitioners to practice using SOAP Notes in real-life situations, building their skills and confidence.

2. **Feedback and Reflection**: Provide regular feedback on documentation practices. Use team meetings to discuss experiences, share best practices, and reflect on areas for improvement.
3. **Ongoing Learning**: Create opportunities for continuous learning, such as workshops and discussion groups. Encourage practitioners to share their experiences and learn from each other.

## Promoting the Use of SOAP Notes

1. **Awareness Campaigns**: Highlight the benefits of using SOAP Notes, such as improved communication, accountability, and ethical decision-making. Use case studies and success stories to illustrate these benefits.
2. **Regular Training**: Offer ongoing training sessions to ensure that all practitioners are familiar with using SOAP Notes. Provide resources and guidelines to support their use.
3. **Recognition**: Recognize and reward practitioners who demonstrate excellence in documentation. Celebrating effective documentation practices encourages others to adopt these methods.

## Resources for Ethics Education and Training

Providing comprehensive and current resources is essential for effective ethics education and training:

1. **Diverse Materials**: Compile a range of resources, including scholarly articles, textbooks, multimedia content, and case studies. These resources should cover foundational ethical principles and specific issues, such as informed consent, end-of-life care, and conflict resolution.
2. **Regular Updates**: Keep training materials up-to-date to reflect the latest research, best practices, and emerging trends. Regular updates ensure that training remains relevant and effective.

3. **Accessibility**: Make resources easily accessible to all staff members. Create a centralized online repository where practitioners can access training materials, guidelines, and case studies.

### Interactive and Engaging Training Methods

Effective training should be interactive and engaging:

1. **Variety of Methods**: Use a mix of teaching methods, including lectures, discussions, case studies, simulations, and role-playing. This variety keeps participants engaged and helps cater to different learning styles.
2. **Real-World Application**: Design training activities that relate to real-world scenarios. Practical exercises that simulate actual ethical dilemmas enhance learning and prepare practitioners for real-life situations.
3. **Feedback and Evaluation**: Encourage participants to provide feedback on training sessions. Use this feedback to refine and improve the training programs, ensuring they meet the needs of the participants.

### Promoting the Use of Educational Resources

1. **Awareness Campaigns**: Develop campaigns to promote the available educational resources. Highlight the importance of continuous learning and how these resources support professional development.
2. **Training and Support**: Provide regular training on how to use the available resources effectively. Offer guidance on how to apply the knowledge gained from these resources to everyday practice.
3. **Recognition**: Acknowledge and reward individuals who actively engage in continuous learning. Recognizing their efforts reinforces the value of ongoing education and encourages others to do the same.

## Conclusion

Practical tools and resources are vital for the effective operation of the Bioethics Program. By using templates, checklists, SOAP Notes, and comprehensive training materials, the director can ensure that policies and procedures align with the program's mission and vision. These tools support the integration of patient autonomy (informed consent), practitioner beneficence (maximize benefits), practitioner nonmaleficence (minimize burdens), and public justice (ensure fairness) into everyday practice, promoting ethical awareness and responsibility. Through structured policy development, thorough documentation, and engaging education, the Bioethics Program can deliver high-quality, ethical patient care and foster a culture of continuous improvement and ethical excellence.

***

The following templates and checklists are designed to support the director in efficiently managing the Bioethics Program and ensuring high standards in policy development, documentation, and ethics education. By using these tools, the director can enhance the consistency, clarity, and effectiveness of the program's processes and initiatives.

***

## 15.1/5.1 Policy Development Template

**Purpose**: To provide a structured and comprehensive framework for developing, implementing, and maintaining clear, legally compliant, and ethically robust policies within the organization.

**Policy Title:** [Title of the Policy]
**Policy Number:** [Assign a unique policy number]
**Date of Creation/Revision:** [Date the policy was created or last revised]
**Effective Date:**[Date the policy comes into effect]
**Review Date:** [Scheduled date for the policy review]

**Purpose**

- Clearly state the purpose of the policy, including its objectives, the issues it addresses, and what it aims to achieve within the organization.

**Scope**

- Define the scope of the policy, including:
  - The individuals, departments, or processes to which the policy applies.
  - Any specific circumstances or contexts under which the policy is applicable.

**Definitions**

- Provide clear definitions for any key terms used within the policy to ensure understanding and consistency in interpretation.

**Policy Statement**

- Articulate the core principles, ethical standards, and key guidelines upon which the policy is based. This section should be a concise declaration of the policy's intentions and overarching framework.

**Procedures**

- Detail the specific steps required to implement and comply with the policy. This should include:
  - **Step-by-Step Guidelines:** A detailed description of the procedures to be followed.
  - **Documentation Requirements:** Outline any forms, checklists, or documentation that must be completed as part of the process.

**Responsibilities**

- Clearly assign and describe the roles and responsibilities of individuals or departments involved in the implementation and oversight of the policy.

**Legal, Ethical, and Compliance Considerations**

- Identify and discuss any relevant laws, regulations, ethical guidelines, or institutional standards that the policy must adhere to. Ensure that the policy aligns with both legal and ethical requirements.

**Training and Education**

- Describe any training or educational initiatives required to effectively implement the policy. Specify the target audience, training content, and delivery methods.

**Monitoring, Compliance, and Evaluation**

- Outline the mechanisms for monitoring adherence to the policy, including:
  - **Compliance Monitoring:** Methods for ensuring that the policy is followed, such as audits or reporting requirements.
  - **Evaluation:** Processes for assessing the effectiveness of the policy and its impact.
  - **Enforcement:** Describe any enforcement actions or consequences for non-compliance.

**Review and Revision Process**

- Detail the process for reviewing and revising the policy, including:

- **Frequency of Review:** How often the policy should be reviewed.
- **Process for Revision:** Steps for making revisions, including who is responsible for the review and how revisions will be approved.

**Related Policies and Documents**

- List any related policies, procedures, or documents that should be consulted in conjunction with this policy to ensure comprehensive coverage of the subject matter.

**Approval**

- Include a section for formal approval, noting the authorities responsible for finalizing and approving the policy.

**Approved by:** [Name and Title]
**Date of Approval:** [Approval Date]

**Appendices**

- Attach or reference any supplementary documents, forms, or additional materials that support the policy.

***

## 15.2/5.2 Policy Development, Review, and Revision Checklist

**Purpose:** To ensure that policies are effectively developed, regularly reviewed, updated, and remain relevant to the organization's goals, compliance requirements, and operational needs.

**Policy Title:** [Title of the Policy]
**Policy Number:** [Policy Number]
**Date:** [Date of Creation/Revision]
**Review Conducted By:** [Name/Title of the Reviewer]
**Next Review Date:** [Scheduled Date of Next Review]

**1. Purpose**

- ☐ Are the policy's objectives clearly stated and aligned with the organization's goals?
- ☐ Does the policy still address a current and relevant issue?

**2. Scope**

- ☐ Is the target audience for the policy clearly defined?
- ☐ Does the policy comprehensively cover all affected parties and situations?

**3. Definitions**

- ☐ Are all key terms clearly defined?
- ☐ Is there consistency with existing policies and terminology?

**4. Procedures**

- ☐ Are the procedures detailed, clear, and practical for implementation?
- ☐ Do the procedures remain applicable and effective?

**5. Responsibilities**

- ☐ Are specific roles and responsibilities clearly assigned?
- ☐ Is accountability for actions and decisions well established?

**6. Compliance and Enforcement**

- ☐ Does the policy comply with current laws, regulations, and ethical guidelines?
- ☐ Are the monitoring and enforcement mechanisms still effective?
- ☐ Are there any consequences for non-compliance outlined clearly?

**7. Effectiveness**

- ☐ Has the policy been effective in achieving its intended outcomes?
- ☐ Are there any gaps, weaknesses, or unintended consequences that need addressing?

**8. Stakeholder Feedback**

- ☐ Has feedback from stakeholders (e.g., practitioners, patients, legal experts) been considered?
- ☐ Have practical challenges identified by stakeholders been addressed?

**9. Training and Implementation**

- ☐ Is additional training or resources required to support the policy's implementation?
- ☐ Are there any barriers to effective implementation that need to be addressed?

**10. References**

- ☐ Are relevant laws, guidelines, and external standards included?
- ☐ Is the policy consistent with external references and internal standards?

**11. Appendices**

- ☐ Are all supplementary materials, forms, and templates attached?

**12. Final Review and Approval**

- ☐ Has the policy been reviewed by all necessary stakeholders?
- ☐ Is the policy ready for approval by the relevant authorities?
- ☐ Are there any additional comments or recommendations for changes to the policy?

**13. Action Taken**

- ☐ Describe any actions taken as a result of the review, including revisions, updates, or the decision to maintain the current policy.

***

## 15.3 SOAP Notes

**Purpose:** To provide a comprehensive and structured format for documenting ethics consultations using the SOAP (Subjective, Objective, Assessment, Plan) method.

**Consultation Date:** [Date]
**Consultant:** [Name/Title]
**Patient/Case ID:** [ID]
**Department:** [Department Name]

### — (S) Subjective

#### Patient's Perspective

- **Narrative**: Document the patient's understanding of their medical condition, goals, values, and concerns.

  **Open-ended Questions:**

  - "Can you tell me about your understanding of your current medical condition?"
  - "What are your goals and priorities regarding your treatment?"
  - "How do you feel about the proposed medical interventions?"
  - "Are there any specific concerns or values that are particularly important to you in making healthcare decisions?"

#### Family's Perspective

- **Narrative**: Document the family's understanding, goals, and concerns regarding the patient's condition and treatment.

  **Open-ended Questions:**

  - "Can you share your thoughts and concerns about your loved one's medical condition and treatment?"
  - "What are your goals and priorities for your loved one's care?"

- "How do you think your loved one feels about their current situation and the proposed treatments?"
- "How do you think your loved one's values and priorities should guide the decisions being made?"

**PRACTITIONERS' PERSPECTIVE**

- **Narrative**: Document the practitioners' views on the medical condition, treatment plan, and ethical considerations.

  **Open-ended Questions:**

  - "Can you explain the medical condition and proposed treatment plan?"
  - "What do you see as the primary benefits and risks of the proposed interventions?"
  - "How do you incorporate the patient's values and preferences into the treatment plan?"
  - "Is the proposed treatment plan in alignment with current healthcare standards of care, institutional policies, and professional guidelines?"
  - "How do you ensure that the treatment plan reflects the patient's reasonable goals, values, and priorities?"

---

## — (O) Objective

**Medical Facts:**

- **Summary**: Provide an overview of the patient's medical condition, diagnosis, and prognosis.
- **Clinical Data**: Include relevant medical history, current treatments, and proposed interventions.
- **Observations**: Note any observations related to the patient's condition and interactions with staff.
- **Alignment**: Ensure that all medical facts align with current medical healthcare standards of care.

## — (A) Assessment

**Ethical Issues Identified:**

- **Patient Autonomy** (informed consent)**:**
  - Assess the patient's capacity to make informed decisions.
  - Document the information provided to the patient about treatment options.
- **Practitioner Beneficence** (promote benefits)**:**
  - Evaluate the potential benefits of the proposed interventions.
- **Practitioner Nonmaleficence** (avoid harm)**:**
  - Identify potential risks and harms associated with the treatments.
- **Public Justice** (promote fairness)**:**
  - Consider fairness in the allocation of resources and treatment options.
- **Alignment with Medical Standards of Care:**
  - Ensure proposed treatment plans adhere to current medical healthcare standards.
- **Patient's Reasonable Goals, Values, and Priorities:**
  - Ensure these are central to the ethical analysis and treatment plan.
- **Compliance with Professional, Institutional, State, and Federal Standards:**
  - Verify that the treatment plan complies with relevant laws, policies, and social expectations.

## — (P) Plan

**Ethical Recommendations**:

- **Steps**: Outline specific steps to address the identified ethical issues.
- **Communication**: Include a plan for further communication with the patient, family, and practitioners.

- **Decisions**: Document any decisions made during the consultation.

**Follow-up:**

- **Meetings**: Schedule follow-up meetings to reassess the situation and ensure implementation of ethical recommendations.
- **Responsibilities**: Assign responsibilities to team members for monitoring the patient's condition and ethical aspects of care.

**Documentation:**

- **EHR**: Ensure all discussions, decisions, and plans are thoroughly documented in the patient's Electronic Health Record (EHR).
- **Alignment**: Confirm that documentation reflects alignment with current healthcare standards, the patient's reasonable goals, values, and priorities, and compliance with professional, institutional, state, and federal standards.

**Signature:** [Consultant's Signature]
**Date:** [Date]

***

## 15.4 Documentation Guidelines

**Purpose**: To provide best practices for accurate and effective documentation of ethics consultations.

**Clarity and Precision**

- Use clear and concise language
- Avoid jargon and technical terms unless necessary
- Ensure that all relevant information is included

**Accuracy**

- Double-check facts and clinical details
- Ensure that patient and case information is correct
- Verify that recommendations align with ethical principles

**Completeness**

- Document all aspects of the consultation, including patient input, clinical observations, and ethical analysis
- Ensure that the plan section includes clear next steps and follow-up actions

**Accessibility**

- Organize notes in a logical order, following the SOAP format
- Ensure that documentation is easily accessible to relevant parties
- Use standardized templates to maintain consistency

**Confidentiality**

- Protect patient privacy by using secure methods for storing and sharing notes
- Only include information that is necessary for the consultation
- Follow institutional guidelines for handling sensitive information

***

# Further Readings and References


## Templates and Checklists for Policy Development

- British Medical Association. (2001). Medical Ethics Today: The BMA's Handbook of Ethics and Law. BMJ Books.
  - *Provides comprehensive templates and checklists for developing and implementing medical ethics policies, essential for bioethics program directors.*
- Clinical Ethics and Policy Group. (2016). Ethical Policy Development and Implementation. University Health Network.
  - *Offers practical guidelines and tools for the development and implementation of ethical policies in healthcare organizations.*

## Sample SOAP Notes and Documentation Guidelines

- Bickley, L. S. (2017). Bates' Guide to Physical Examination and History Taking (12th ed.). Wolters Kluwer.
  - *Includes detailed instructions and examples of SOAP Notes, providing essential documentation guidelines for clinical and ethics consultations.*
- Pomerantz, W. J., & Schafermeyer, R. (2002). SOAP documentation. Emergency Medicine Clinics of North America, 20(1), 165-174.
  - *Examines best practices for SOAP documentation, offering practical guidance for accurate and effective record-keeping in emergency and clinical settings.*

## Resources for Ethics Education and Training

- Pellegrino, E. D., & Thomasma, D. C. (1993). The Virtues in Medical Practice. Oxford University Press.
  - *Discusses the virtues essential to medical practice and their role in ethics education and training for healthcare professionals.*

- Roberts, L. W., & Dyer, A. R. (Eds.). (2004). Concise Guide to Ethics in Mental Health Care. American Psychiatric Publishing.
  - *Provides a concise yet comprehensive guide to ethics in mental health care, useful for ethics education and training programs.*

***

# Chapter 16: Case Studies and Clinical Vignettes

Case studies and clinical vignettes are instrumental tools for illustrating complex ethical dilemmas and enhancing the understanding and application of ethical principles in clinical practice. By analyzing real-world examples, practitioners can engage in reflective discussions, develop their ethical reasoning skills, and apply ethical principles to their own practice. This chapter provides guidance on incorporating case studies into the Bioethics Program, ensuring alignment with the program's mission and vision by focusing on patient autonomy (informed consent), practitioner beneficence (maximize benefits), practitioner nonmaleficence (minimize burdens), and public justice (ensure fairness). These case studies also support compliance with institutional policies, established medical standards of care, and legal mandates.

## The Value of Real-world Examples of Complex Ethical Dilemmas

Real-world examples provide a tangible context for understanding and applying the core bioethical principles. They illustrate the complexities and nuances of ethical dilemmas, highlighting the challenges and considerations involved in ethical decision-making. By examining these cases, practitioners gain a deeper understanding of the ethical issues they may encounter in their practice and develop strategies for addressing them effectively.

1. **Patient Autonomy** (Informed Consent): Case studies should emphasize the patient's right to informed consent and decision-making. These cases should demonstrate how practitioners can ensure that patients or their surrogates understand their diagnosis and prognosis, are aware of all available treatment

options, comprehend the purpose of each option, and can assess the potential benefits and risks.

2. **Practitioner Beneficence** (Maximize Benefits): Real-world cases can illustrate how practitioners can maximize the benefits to patients, promoting their well-being based on the patient's reasonable goals, values, and priorities. These cases highlight the importance of aligning treatment options with what is beneficial for the patient, compliant with medical standards of care, institutional policies, and legal mandates all while considering the patient's reasonable goals, values and priorities.
3. **Practitioner Beneficence** (Minimize Burdens): Case studies can show how to avoid unnecessary harm or risks to the patient. These examples can be used to discuss scenarios where the potential for harm must be minimized, illustrating the delicate balance between providing beneficial interventions and minimize burdens.
4. **Public Justice** (Ensure Fairness): By including examples that address fairness and equitable treatment, case studies can explore the broader implications of healthcare decisions on society. These cases provide insights into how decisions should align with ethical standards, institutional policies, and legal requirements to promote fairness.

## Incorporating Case Studies into Training

The director should integrate case studies into various training formats, including workshops, ethics rounds, and interactive sessions. These activities provide a forum for discussing and reflecting on ethical dilemmas, allowing practitioners to develop their ethical reasoning skills and apply ethical principles to real-world scenarios:

1. **Workshops and Seminars:** Incorporate case studies into the curriculum to facilitate discussions around ethical issues. These sessions can involve group work, presentations, and role-playing to engage participants actively.

2. **Ethics Rounds**: Use case studies in ethics rounds to provide a structured way of exploring ethical dilemmas. These discussions can involve interprofessional teams, offering different perspectives and fostering comprehensive ethical analysis.
3. **Interactive Learning**: Develop online modules and simulations based on real-world case studies. These tools can provide flexible and accessible learning opportunities, allowing practitioners to explore ethical scenarios at their own pace.

## Promoting the Use of Case Studies

To maximize their impact, the director should actively promote the use of case studies within the organization:

1. **Awareness Campaigns**: Create campaigns highlighting the importance of case studies in ethical education. Share success stories where case studies have led to improved ethical decision-making.
2. **Training and Support**: Provide regular training on how to use case studies effectively. Offer resources, guidelines, and examples to help practitioners incorporate case studies into their learning and practice.
3. **Recognition**: Recognize and celebrate practitioners who effectively use case studies to enhance their ethical practice. Acknowledgment of good practice encourages others to adopt these methods.

## Interprofessional Approach to Ethics Education

Analyzing cases from various medical specialties provides a comprehensive understanding of the ethical issues that can arise in different contexts. The director should include case studies from specialties such as oncology, pediatrics, psychiatry, and surgery, highlighting the unique ethical challenges and considerations in each field:

1. **Oncology**: Case studies in oncology can explore issues related to end-of-life care, informed consent, and palliative care. These

cases often involve complex decisions about treatment options, quality of life, and patient autonomy.

2. **Pediatrics**: Pediatric cases can focus on issues such as parental consent, best interests of the child, and decisional capacity of minors. These cases provide insights into balancing the rights of parents and the needs of the child.
3. **Psychiatry**: Ethical dilemmas in psychiatry may involve patient autonomy, confidentiality, and involuntary treatment. These cases can highlight the challenges of respecting patient rights while ensuring safety and well-being.
4. **Surgery**: Surgical cases can explore issues related to risk, informed consent, and the ethics of elective procedures. These scenarios can illustrate the importance of clear communication and shared decision-making.

## Facilitating Discussions and Reflections

The director should facilitate discussions and reflections on case studies from various medical specialties. These activities provide opportunities for practitioners to explore ethical principles, decision-making frameworks, and practical considerations:

1. **Structured Discussions**: Use a structured format for discussing case studies, such as guided questions or ethical analysis frameworks. This approach helps participants focus on key issues and develop their ethical reasoning skills.
2. **Reflective Practice**: Encourage practitioners to reflect on their experiences and share insights gained from analyzing case studies. Reflection helps deepen understanding and reinforces the application of ethical principles.
3. **Interdisciplinary Collaboration**: Promote interdisciplinary discussions to bring diverse perspectives to the analysis of case studies. This collaboration enriches the learning experience and provides a broader understanding of ethical issues.

**Promoting the Use of Interprofessional Case Studies**:

To maximize the benefits of interprofessional case studies, the director should actively promote their use:

1. **Incorporate in Training**: Make interprofessional case studies a core component of ethics training programs. Use these cases to highlight the relevance of ethical principles across different medical specialties.
2. **Develop Resources**: Create a repository of case studies from various specialties. Make these resources easily accessible to practitioners for use in training and ethics rounds.
3. **Encourage Collaboration**: Foster a culture of collaboration by encouraging practitioners from different specialties to work together on case study analysis. This collaboration helps build a comprehensive understanding of ethical issues.

## Lessons Learned and Best Practices

Lessons learned and best practices provide valuable insights for addressing ethical dilemmas and enhancing ethical practice. The director should compile and share lessons learned from real-world cases, highlighting key takeaways and strategies that can be applied to future situations:

1. **Effective Communication:** Highlight the importance of clear, honest, and compassionate communication with patients and families. Lessons learned can provide examples of how effective communication can resolve ethical conflicts and build trust.
2. **Conflict Resolution**: Share strategies for managing and resolving conflicts that arise during ethics consultations. Best practices can include techniques for mediation, negotiation, and finding common ground.
3. **Ethical Analysis and Decision-making**: Provide insights into effective ethical analysis and decision-making processes. This can include the use of decision-making frameworks, ethical principles, and consultation with ethics committees.

## Staying Informed About Emerging Trends

To ensure the Bioethics Program remains relevant and effective, the director should stay informed about emerging trends in the field of bioethics:

1. **Professional Development**: Attend professional conferences, participate in training programs, and engage with professional organizations to stay updated on the latest developments in bioethics.
2. **Continuous Improvement**: Incorporate new insights, research findings, and best practices into the Bioethics Program. Continuous improvement ensures that the program remains dynamic and responsive to the needs of the organization.
3. **Networking and Collaboration**: Build relationships with other bioethics professionals and organizations. Collaboration provides opportunities to share knowledge, learn from others, and stay at the forefront of bioethical practice.

## Promoting a Culture of Continuous Learning

To maximize the impact of lessons learned and best practices, the director should foster a culture of continuous learning:

1. **Create Learning Opportunities**: Develop forums, workshops, and discussion groups where practitioners can share experiences, learn from each other, and discuss ethical dilemmas.
2. **Encourage Reflection**: Promote reflective practice by encouraging practitioners to think about their experiences, identify lessons learned, and apply them to future situations.
3. **Recognize and Celebrate Success**: Acknowledge and reward practitioners who demonstrate a commitment to continuous learning and ethical excellence. Celebrating success reinforces the value of ethical practice and encourages others to strive for excellence.

## Conclusion

Case studies and clinical vignettes are powerful tools for enhancing the Bioethics Program's effectiveness. By integrating real-world examples, interprofessional cases, lessons learned, and best practices, the director can support the development of ethical reasoning skills, promote ethical decision-making, and ensure alignment with the program's mission and vision. These tools not only enrich ethics education and training but also enhance the overall quality of patient care by embedding ethical principles into clinical practice. Through continuous learning and reflection, the Bioethics Program can foster a culture of ethical awareness, responsibility, and compassion, ultimately leading to the maximization of patient well-being and the promotion of justice and fairness in healthcare.

***

The following templates will assist the Bioethics Program Director in systematically documenting, analyzing, and discussing ethical dilemmas, while also capturing and sharing lessons learned to foster continuous improvement within the program.

***

## 16.1 Case Study Template

**Purpose**: To provide a structured format for documenting and analyzing real-world ethical dilemmas in clinical practice.

**Title**: [Case Title]
**Date**: [Date]
**Medical Specialty**: [e.g., Oncology, Pediatrics, Psychiatry]

**Background:**

- **Patient Information**: [Age, gender, medical history, etc.]
- **Clinical Context**: [Describe the medical condition and treatment options]
- **Ethical Dilemma**: [Detail the ethical issue(s) encountered]

**Key Ethical Principles Involved:**

- **Patient Autonomy** (Informed Consent): [Description of how patient autonomy is involved]
- **Beneficence** (Maximize Benefits): [Description of how beneficence is involved]
- **Nonmaleficence** (Minimize Burdens): [Description of how nonmaleficence is involved]
- **Justice** (Ensure Fairness): [Description of how justice is involved]

**Decision-Making Process:**

- **Stakeholders**: [List the individuals or groups involved]
- **Discussion**: [Summarize the ethical discussions and considerations]
- **Resolution**: [Describe the final decision and rationale]

**Outcome:**

- **Short-Term**: [Immediate outcomes of the decision]
- **Long-Term**: [Long-term impacts on the patient, family, and healthcare team]

**Lessons Learned:**

- **Key Takeaways**: [Summarize the main lessons learned from this case]
- **Best Practices**: [List any best practices identified]

**References:**

- **Citations**: [List any references used in the case study]

***

## 16.2 Clinical Vignette Template

**Purpose**: To create a concise summary of a clinical scenario that can be used for training and discussion purposes.

**Title**: [Vignette Title]
**Date**: [Date]
**Medical Specialty**: [e.g., Surgery, Emergency Medicine, Palliative Care]

**Scenario Overview:**

- **Patient Background**: [Brief description of the patient's condition and history]
- **Clinical Situation**: [Summary of the clinical situation or event]
- **Ethical Issue**: [Identify the primary ethical dilemma or conflict]

**Ethical Analysis:**

- **Ethical Principles**: [Discuss how the key ethical principles apply to this scenario]
- **Stakeholder Perspectives**: [Summarize the views and concerns of the involved parties]

**Proposed Solutions:**

- **Options**: [List the possible courses of action]
- **Recommendations**: [Provide a recommended course of action with justification]

**Discussion Questions:**

- **For Group Reflection**: [List questions to guide group discussion and analysis]
- **For Individual Reflection**: [List questions for personal reflection and ethical reasoning]

***

## 16.3 Lessons Learned and Best Practices Summary

**Purpose**: To capture and share key takeaways and best practices from analyzed cases, ensuring continuous improvement in ethical decision-making.

**Title**: [Summary Title]
**Date**: [Date]

**Case(s) Analyzed:**

- **Case Title 1**: [Brief description and key ethical issues]
- **Case Title 2**: [Brief description and key ethical issues]

**Key Lessons Learned:**

- **Lesson 1**: [Summarize a significant lesson learned]
- **Lesson 2**: [Summarize another significant lesson learned]

**Best Practices Identified:**

- **Best Practice 1**: [Describe a best practice identified from the case(s)]
- **Best Practice 2**: [Describe another best practice]

**Recommendations for Implementation:**

- **Strategy 1**: [Outline a strategy for implementing best practices]
- **Strategy 2**: [Outline another implementation strategy]

**Next Steps:**

- **Action Plan**: [Describe any planned actions based on the lessons learned and best practices]
- **Follow-Up**: [Detail any follow-up required to assess the impact of implemented practices]

***

## Further Readings and References

### Real-world Examples of Complex Ethical Dilemmas


- Jonsen, A. R., Siegler, M., & Winslade, W. J. (2010). Clinical Ethics: A Practical Approach to Ethical Decisions in Clinical Medicine (7th ed.). McGraw-Hill Education.
  - *Offers practical examples of complex ethical dilemmas in clinical medicine, providing valuable insights and case studies for ethics consultations.*
- Rhodes, R., & Alfandre, D. (2007). A systematic approach to clinical moral reasoning. Clinical Ethics, 2(2), 66-70.
  - *Presents a structured approach to clinical moral reasoning, illustrated with real-world case studies to enhance understanding of ethical decision-making.*


### Analyzing Cases from Various Medical Specialties


- Faden, R. R., Beauchamp, T. L., & King, N. M. P. (1986). A History and Theory of Informed Consent. Oxford University Press.
  - *Provides historical and theoretical perspectives on informed consent, including case analyses from various medical specialties.*
- Moreno, J. D. (2005). Is There an Ethicist in the House? On the Cutting Edge of Bioethics. Indiana University Press.
  - *Explores contemporary issues in bioethics through case studies, offering insights into the ethical challenges faced across different medical specialties.*


### Lessons Learned and Best Practices


- Childress, J. F. (2007). Public Bioethics: Principles and Problems. Oxford University Press.
  - *Discusses principles and problems in public bioethics, highlighting lessons learned and best practices for addressing ethical issues.*

- Pellegrino, E. D., & Thomasma, D. C. (1993). The Virtues in Medical Practice. Oxford University Press.
    - *Emphasizes the importance of virtues in medical practice, providing best practices for ethical conduct and decision-making.*

***

# Chapter 17: The Future of Bioethics Program Leadership

As the healthcare landscape evolves, so too must the Bioethics Program adapt to meet new challenges and opportunities. This chapter focuses on the future of bioethics leadership, emphasizing the integration of core bioethical principles—patient autonomy (informed consent), practitioner beneficence (maximize benefits), practitioner nonmaleficence (minimize burdens), and public justice (ensure fairness)—into emerging contexts. The director must remain vigilant, informed, and responsive to ensure the Bioethics Program remains relevant, effective, and aligned with institutional policies, established medical standards of care, and legal mandates.

## Staying Informed About Emerging Ethical Issues

The field of bioethics is constantly evolving, with new challenges and opportunities emerging due to advancements in technology, changes in healthcare regulations, and shifts in societal values. The director must stay informed about these developments and be prepared to address new ethical issues as they arise. By remaining informed and adaptable, the director can ensure that the Bioethics Program continues to support ethical decision-making in a changing healthcare environment.

- **Monitoring Trends**: The director should regularly review academic literature, participate in professional networks, and engage with bioethics organizations to stay updated on emerging ethical issues.
- **Engaging with Experts**: Collaborating with experts in emerging fields such as biotechnology, artificial intelligence, and data ethics can provide valuable insights into the ethical challenges posed by new technologies and practices.

- **Proactive Adaptation**: The director should establish protocols for integrating new ethical considerations into the Bioethics Program. This might include developing new policies, updating training programs, and revising consultation procedures to address emerging issues.

## Navigating Emerging Technologies

Technological advancements present both ethical challenges and opportunities. Technologies such as artificial intelligence, genetic engineering, and telemedicine are reshaping healthcare delivery, raising critical ethical questions that must be addressed.

- **Artificial Intelligence (AI)**: AI technologies can enhance healthcare by improving diagnostic accuracy and treatment personalization. However, they also raise concerns about patient autonomy, data privacy, and the potential for bias in decision-making algorithms. The director should guide the integration of AI in ways that respect patient rights, ensure transparency, and promote fairness.
- **Genetic Engineering**: Advances in genetic engineering, such as CRISPR, offer promising treatments for genetic disorders but also pose ethical dilemmas related to human enhancement, consent, and the potential long-term effects on the human gene pool. The director should develop guidelines to navigate these ethical issues, balancing innovation with ethical responsibility.
- **Telemedicine**: The expansion of telemedicine has improved access to healthcare, especially during the COVID-19 pandemic. However, it also presents challenges related to informed consent, privacy, and the quality of patient-practitioner interactions. The director should ensure that telemedicine practices adhere to ethical standards, safeguarding patient autonomy and confidentiality.

## Adapting to Changes in Healthcare Regulations

Healthcare regulations are continually evolving, influencing ethical considerations in clinical practice. The director must stay informed about regulatory changes and be prepared to adapt the Bioethics Program accordingly.

- **Regulatory Updates**: The director should subscribe to updates from regulatory bodies, attend legal seminars, and engage with healthcare compliance experts to stay informed about changes in regulations.
- **Policy Revisions**: When regulations change, the director must review and update the Bioethics Program's policies to ensure compliance. This may include revising guidelines for informed consent, patient confidentiality, and data security.
- **Training and Education**: The director should provide ongoing training to practitioners about new regulations and their ethical implications. This training ensures that all staff members understand their ethical responsibilities and are equipped to comply with legal requirements.

## Addressing Evolving Societal Values

Societal values are not static; they evolve over time, influenced by cultural, social, and political factors. These changes impact ethical decision-making in healthcare, requiring the Bioethics Program to be responsive and adaptable.

- **Cultural Sensitivity**: The director should promote a culture of respect for diverse values and beliefs. This involves incorporating cultural competence into ethics training and ensuring that ethics consultations are sensitive to the cultural and personal values of patients.
- **Community Engagement**: Engaging with the community through forums, surveys, and public discussions can provide insights into evolving societal values. The director should use this feedback to inform the Bioethics Program's approach to ethical issues.
- **Ethical Reflection**: Encouraging continuous ethical reflection among practitioners helps them remain sensitive to changes in

societal values. This reflection can be facilitated through discussion groups, case studies, and ethics rounds.

### Expanding the Scope and Reach of the Bioethics Program

The director should explore opportunities to expand the Bioethics Program's scope and reach, integrating ethical considerations into new areas of practice, such as public health, community health, and global health.

- **Public Health Ethics**: Ethical issues in public health, such as vaccination mandates, health surveillance, and pandemic response, require careful consideration. The director should incorporate public health ethics into the Bioethics Program, providing guidance on balancing individual rights with public welfare.
- **Community Health**: Addressing social determinants of health, health disparities, and access to care are critical ethical issues in community health. The director should work with community leaders and health organizations to promote ethical practices that address these challenges.
- **Global Health**: Ethical issues in global health include equitable access to healthcare resources, medical research ethics, and the impact of globalization on health. The director should collaborate with international bioethics organizations to ensure that the Bioethics Program considers global ethical standards and practices.

### Promoting a Culture of Ethical Awareness and Responsibility

The director should actively promote a culture of ethical awareness and responsibility throughout the organization.

- **Awareness Campaigns**: Develop campaigns that highlight the importance of ethics in healthcare, showcasing ethical success stories and promoting ethical behavior.

- **Regular Training and Support**: Offer continuous training opportunities that emphasize the importance of ethical decision-making. This training should be accessible to all staff members, from frontline healthcare workers to administrative personnel.
- **Recognizing Ethical Behavior**: Establish programs to recognize and reward ethical behavior within the organization. Acknowledging those who demonstrate ethical leadership reinforces the importance of ethics and inspires others to follow suit.

## Leading the Evolution of Bioethics in Healthcare

As the role of bioethics continues to evolve, the director should be prepared to lead this evolution, ensuring that ethical considerations remain at the forefront of healthcare delivery.

- **Thought Leadership**: The director should contribute to the broader field of bioethics by publishing research, participating in academic conferences, and engaging with professional bioethics organizations.
- **Organizational Leadership**: Within the organization, the director should lead by example, demonstrating a commitment to ethical excellence. This involves mentoring others, advocating for ethical practices, and fostering an environment where ethical issues are openly discussed and addressed.
- **Advocacy**: The director should advocate for the integration of ethical considerations into all aspects of healthcare delivery, from clinical practice to organizational policies. By championing the importance of ethics, the director can help shape a healthcare system that values integrity, compassion, and justice.

## Final Thoughts on Leading with Integrity and Compassion

### Modeling Ethical Behavior

The director should model ethical behavior in all interactions and decisions. This involves demonstrating integrity, empathy, and compassion in dealings with patients, families, colleagues, and the broader community. By modeling ethical behavior, the director sets a standard for others to follow, fostering a culture of ethical awareness and responsibility.

### Communicating Openly and Honestly

Open and honest communication is essential for building trust and credibility. The director should communicate transparently with all stakeholders, providing clear information about ethical issues and decision-making processes. By fostering open communication, the director builds trust, supports collaboration, and enhances the Bioethics Program's effectiveness.

### Treating All Stakeholders with Respect and Dignity

Respect and dignity are fundamental principles of ethical leadership. The director should treat all stakeholders—patients, families, healthcare providers, and community members—with respect, recognizing their unique perspectives and contributions. By valuing and respecting others, the director can build positive relationships, enhance collaboration, and strengthen the Bioethics Program's impact.

### Inspiring Others

Leadership in bioethics is not only about making ethical decisions but also about inspiring others to do the same. The director should articulate a compelling vision for the Bioethics Program, one that emphasizes the importance of ethics in healthcare and inspires others to uphold ethical principles. By leading with integrity and compassion, the director can inspire a commitment to ethical excellence, ensuring that the Bioethics Program continues to support the delivery of high-quality, ethical patient care.

## A Vision for the Future

The future of bioethics lies in the hands of dedicated leaders who are committed to ethical excellence and continuous improvement. By embracing their role in shaping the ethical landscape of healthcare, these leaders can create a legacy of ethical practice that benefits patients, healthcare providers, and society at large. The Bioethics Program will continue to evolve, addressing new challenges and opportunities as they arise. Through thoughtful leadership, ongoing education, and a commitment to the core principles of bioethics, the program will remain a vital component of ethical healthcare delivery. As we look to the future, let us commit to leading with integrity, compassion, and a steadfast dedication to ethical excellence.

***

The following forms and templates are designed to assist the Bioethics Program Director in navigating emerging challenges, ensuring compliance with regulations, engaging stakeholders effectively, and leading with integrity and compassion. They provide practical tools to support the continuous improvement of the Bioethics Program and the professional growth of its leadership.

***

## 17.1 Emerging Technologies Ethical Impact Assessment Template

**Purpose**: To evaluate the ethical implications of new technologies and guide decision-making within the Bioethics Program.

**Technology Name**: [Name of the technology]
**Date**: [Date]

**Overview:**

- **Description of Technology**: [Provide a brief overview of the technology]
- **Current and Potential Applications**: [List the applications of the technology in healthcare]
- **Stakeholders Involved**: [Identify key stakeholders impacted by this technology]

**Ethical Considerations:**

- **Patient Autonomy** (Informed Consent): [Discuss how the technology impacts patient autonomy]
- **Beneficence** (Maximize Benefits) **and Nonmaleficence** (Minimize Burdens): [Evaluate the potential benefits and harms]
- **Justice** (Ensure Fairness): [Consider how the technology affects fairness and equality]
- **Privacy and Confidentiality**: [Analyze the impact on patient privacy and data protection]

**Regulatory and Legal Concerns:**

- **Current Regulations**: [List relevant laws and regulations]
- **Compliance Requirements**: [Identify any compliance needs]
- **Potential Legal Risks**: [Describe any legal risks associated with the technology]

**Recommendations:**

- **Ethical Guidelines**: [Provide recommendations for ethical use]
- **Implementation Strategies**: [Outline steps for integrating the technology ethically]
- **Monitoring and Evaluation**: [Suggest methods for ongoing assessment of ethical impact]

**Conclusion:**

- **Summary of Findings**: [Summarize key findings from the assessment]
- **Next Steps**: [List any actions to be taken based on the assessment]

***

## 17.2 Regulatory Changes Adaptation Plan Template

**Purpose**: To help the Bioethics Program adapt to changes in healthcare regulations by outlining a clear plan of action.

**Regulation Name**: [Name of the regulation]
**Effective Date**: [Date]

**Summary of Changes:**

- **Description of Regulatory Change**: [Provide a brief overview of the regulation]
- **Implications for Bioethics Program**: [Describe how the regulation impacts the program]
- **Key Stakeholders**: [Identify who is affected by the change]

**Action Plan:**

- **Assessment of Current Compliance**: [Evaluate current compliance status]
- **Required Adjustments**: [List the changes needed to comply with the new regulation]
- **Responsible Parties**: [Assign tasks to specific team members or departments]
- **Timeline**: [Provide a timeline for implementation]
- **Resources Needed**: [Identify any resources required to implement changes]

**Training and Communication:**

- **Staff Training Plan**: [Outline the training plan for staff on the new regulation]
- **Communication Strategy**: [Describe how the changes will be communicated to stakeholders]
- **Feedback Mechanisms**: [Provide a way to gather feedback from stakeholders]

**Monitoring and Evaluation:**

- **Compliance Checks**: [Set up regular checks to ensure compliance]
- **Review Process**: [Establish a process for ongoing review and adjustment]
- **Reporting**: [Outline how progress and issues will be reported]

**Conclusion:**

- **Summary of Plan**: [Summarize the adaptation plan]
- **Next Steps**: [List any follow-up actions required]

***

## 17.3 Stakeholder Engagement Plan Template

**Purpose**: To ensure effective engagement with stakeholders in addressing evolving societal values and promoting a culture of ethical awareness.

**Project/Initiative Name**: [Name of the project or initiative]
**Date**: [Date]

**Objective:**

- **Purpose of Engagement**: [State the purpose of engaging with stakeholders]
- **Goals**: [List the goals of stakeholder engagement]

**Stakeholder Identification:**

- **Key Stakeholders**: [Identify the primary stakeholders]
- **Roles and Interests**: [Describe the roles and interests of each stakeholder group]
- **Potential Concerns**: [List any concerns or issues that stakeholders may have]

**Engagement Strategy:**

- **Methods of Engagement**: [Describe how stakeholders will be engaged (e.g., meetings, surveys, forums)]
- **Frequency**: [Specify how often engagement activities will occur]
- **Communication Channels**: [List the communication channels to be used]

**Key Messages:**

- **Core Messages**: [Outline the key messages to communicate to stakeholders]
- **Tailored Messaging**: [Provide specific messages for different stakeholder groups]

**Feedback and Evaluation:**

- **Feedback Mechanisms**: [Describe how feedback will be collected and used]
- **Evaluation Criteria**: [Set criteria for evaluating the effectiveness of stakeholder engagement]
- **Adjustments and Follow-Up**: [Plan for making adjustments based on feedback]

**Conclusion:**

- **Summary of Plan**: [Summarize the stakeholder engagement plan]
- **Next Steps**: [List any follow-up actions required]

***

## Further Readings and References


- Jonsen, A. R., Siegler, M., & Winslade, W. J. (2010). Clinical Ethics: A Practical Approach to Ethical Decisions in Clinical Medicine (7th ed.). McGraw-Hill Education.
    - *Discusses the future directions of clinical ethics, offering practical approaches to ethical decision-making in evolving medical contexts.*
- Rhodes, R., & Alfandre, D. (2007). A systematic approach to clinical moral reasoning. Clinical Ethics, 2(2), 66-70.
    - *Explores future trends in clinical moral reasoning, emphasizing systematic approaches to evolving ethical challenges.*
- Faden, R. R., Beauchamp, T. L., & King, N. M. P. (1986). A History and Theory of Informed Consent. Oxford University Press.
    - *Provides foundational insights into the future of informed consent, considering historical and theoretical developments.*
- Moreno, J. D. (2005). Is There an Ethicist in the House? On the Cutting Edge of Bioethics. Indiana University Press.
    - *Examines the future of bioethics through cutting-edge issues and challenges, offering a forward-looking perspective.*
- Childress, J. F. (2007). Public Bioethics: Principles and Problems. Oxford University Press.
    - *Analyzes future trends and challenges in public bioethics, offering principles and solutions for emerging ethical issues.*
- Pellegrino, E. D., & Thomasma, D. C. (1993). The Virtues in Medical Practice. Oxford University Press.
    - *Discusses the role of virtues in the future of medical practice, providing insights into ethical leadership and decision-making.*

- Covey, S. R., & Merrill, R. R. (2006). The Speed of Trust: The One Thing That Changes Everything. Free Press.
  - *Explores the critical role of trust in future organizational success, emphasizing strategies for building and maintaining trust.*
- Mayer, R. C., Davis, J. H., & Schoorman, F. D. (1995). An integrative model of organizational trust. Academy of Management Review, 20(3), 709-734.
  - *Offers an integrative model of organizational trust, highlighting its importance for future bioethics program leadership.*
- Kouzes, J. M., & Posner, B. Z. (2017). The Leadership Challenge: How to Make Extraordinary Things Happen in Organizations (6th ed.). Wiley.
  - *Provides insights into the future of leadership, emphasizing the importance of leading by example and inspiring others in the field of bioethics.*
- Burns, J. M. (1978). Leadership. Harper & Row.
  - *A seminal work on leadership, discussing the transformative power of leadership and its role in shaping the future of bioethics programs.*


***

# Review Questions

**True/False Questions:**

1. Templates and checklists can enhance the quality and consistency of bioethics policies.
True or False?

2. SOAP Notes are used to document the patient's narrative, clinical findings, ethical analysis, and planned actions.
True or False?

3. Regular training is not necessary for practitioners to effectively use SOAP Notes in ethics consultations.
True or False?

4. Comprehensive documentation helps in building trust and credibility within the organization.
True or False?

5. Including real-world examples in training sessions does not contribute significantly to understanding ethical dilemmas.
True or False?

**Multiple-Choice Questions:**

6. What is a key benefit of using templates for policy development in bioethics programs?
a) They allow for more flexibility and less structure
b) They reduce the need for regular reviews
c) They ensure policies are clear, consistent, and comprehensive
d) They eliminate the need for practitioner training

7. What is one of the main sections in a well-structured policy document?
a) Financial statements
b) Personal anecdotes
c) Scope and definitions
d) Marketing strategies

**Clinical Vignettes:**

8. A hospital ethics committee is drafting a new policy on end-of-life care. What should be included to ensure clarity and effectiveness?
a) Personal opinions of the committee members
b) Detailed procedures and assigned responsibilities
c) Minimal guidelines to allow flexibility
d) Irrelevant historical data

9. During an ethics consultation, a healthcare provider struggles to document the ethical analysis accurately. What is the best course of action?
a) Ignore the inaccuracies and proceed
b) Provide additional training and support for accurate documentation
c) Assign the documentation task to another practitioner
d) Discontinue using SOAP Notes

10. A new practitioner is unsure how to use the organization's documentation guidelines effectively. What should the Bioethics Program Director do?
a) Ignore the practitioner's concerns
b) Offer targeted training sessions and mentorship
c) Replace the practitioner with someone more experienced
d) Simplify the guidelines to avoid confusion

## Correct Answers:

1. True
2. True
3. False (Regular training is necessary for practitioners to effectively use SOAP Notes in ethics consultations.)
4. True
5. False (Including real-world examples in training sessions does contribute significantly to understanding ethical dilemmas.)
6. c) They ensure policies are clear, consistent, and comprehensive
7. c) Scope and definitions
8. b) Detailed procedures and assigned responsibilities
9. b) Provide additional training and support for accurate documentation
10. b) Offer targeted training sessions and mentorship

***

# Appendix:

## Templates, Checklists, and Assessments

In this appendix, you will find a comprehensive list of the forms, templates, checklists, and assessments referenced throughout the text. Each item is presented with its title and purpose, providing you with a clear understanding of its role and relevance within the broader context of the Bioethics Program.

**Purpose and Use:** This appendix serves as a practical guide, allowing you to quickly identify and locate the specific tools you need for various aspects of ethics consultation, leadership, policy development, and more. By understanding the purpose of each tool, you can better utilize them to enhance the quality and effectiveness of your ethical decision-making processes, training programs, and organizational practices.

**How to Use This Appendix**:

- **Reference Guide:** Use this appendix as a quick reference to find the appropriate tools for different stages of the ethics consultation process, policy development, and other related activities.
- **Implementation:** Refer to the corresponding sections in the text for detailed instructions on how to implement and customize these tools for your specific needs.
- **Customization:** Consider how each tool can be adapted to fit the unique requirements of your organization, ensuring that they align with your goals and ethical standards.
- **Training and Development:** Incorporate these tools into your ethics training programs and professional development initiatives to promote consistent and ethical practices across your organization.

By leveraging the resources in this appendix, you can ensure that your Bioethics Program operates with the highest standards of clarity, accountability, and ethical integrity.

---

## I. Leadership and Strategy

**14.1 Stakeholder Trust-Building Checklist**
Purpose: To ensure that the director is consistently taking actions to build and maintain trust with stakeholders.

**1.1 Bioethics Leadership Self-Assessment Tool**
Purpose: To help the Bioethics Program Director regularly assess their ethical leadership practices, competencies, and identify areas for personal and professional growth.

**1.3 Ethics Program Development Checklist**
Purpose: To guide the Bioethics Program Director through the essential steps of developing or refining a Bioethics Program, ensuring that all critical elements are addressed.

**2.1 Strategic Alignment Checklist**
Purpose: To ensure that the Bioethics Program aligns with the organization's strategic goals and objectives.

**3.1 Mission Statement Development Template**
Purpose: To guide the development of a clear and concise Mission Statement for the Bioethics Program.

**3.2 Vision Statement Development Template**
Purpose: To outline the long-term goals and aspirations of the Bioethics Program, ensuring alignment with the organization's ethical commitments.

**3.3 Values Statement Development Template**
Purpose: To articulate the core ethical principles that will guide the Bioethics Program's actions and decision-making processes.

**3.4 Communication Plan Template**
Purpose: To create a structured plan for communicating the

Mission, Vision, and Values of the Bioethics Program to stakeholders.

**1.4 Stakeholder Engagement Template**
Purpose: To plan and track engagement with key stakeholders, ensuring that their perspectives are considered in bioethics program decisions and initiatives.

**17.3 Stakeholder Engagement Plan Template**
Purpose: To ensure effective engagement with stakeholders in addressing evolving societal values and promoting a culture of ethical awareness.

**17.2 Regulatory Changes Adaptation Plan Template**
Purpose: To help the Bioethics Program adapt to changes in healthcare regulations by outlining a clear plan of action.

**1.5 Bioethics Program Director's Monthly Report Template**
Purpose: To document and report on the monthly activities, challenges, and achievements of the Bioethics Program, ensuring accountability and transparency.

**14.2 Recognition and Inspiration Log**
Purpose: To track efforts to recognize team members and inspire ethical practices within the Bioethics Program.

---

## II. Program Development and Documentation

**15.1/5.1 Policy Development Template**
Purpose: To provide a structured and comprehensive framework for developing, implementing, and maintaining clear, legally compliant, and ethically robust policies within the organization.

**15.2/5.2 Policy Development Checklist**
Purpose: To ensure that policies are effectively developed, regularly reviewed, updated, and remain relevant to the organization's goals, compliance requirements, and operational needs.

**5.4 Informed Consent Policy Template**
Purpose: To provide a clear and comprehensive template for developing a policy on informed consent, ensuring that all legal, ethical, and practical considerations are addressed.

**5.3 Policy Implementation and Communication**
Purpose: To outline the steps required to effectively communicate and implement a new or revised policy within the organization.

**5.5 Policy Feedback Form**
Purpose: To gather continuous feedback from practitioners on the effectiveness and practicality of existing policies.

**1.2 Ethical Dilemma Case Documentation Form**
Purpose: To document ethical dilemmas encountered in the healthcare setting, ensuring that they are analyzed, resolved, and reviewed systematically.

**16.1 Case Study Template**
Purpose: To provide a structured format for documenting and analyzing real-world ethical dilemmas in clinical practice.

**16.2 Clinical Vignette Template**
Purpose: To create a concise summary of a clinical scenario that can be used for training and discussion purposes.

**16.3 Lessons Learned and Best Practices Summary**
Purpose: To capture and share key takeaways and best practices from analyzed cases, ensuring continuous improvement in ethical decision-making.

---

## III. Ethics Consultation Tools

**4.1 Structured Process for Ethics Consultations**
Purpose: To provide a comprehensive and systematic framework for conducting healthcare ethics consultations with clarity, transparency, and empathy, while promoting continuous improvement and ethical excellence.

**4.2 SOAP Notes**

Purpose: To provide a comprehensive and structured format for documenting ethics consultations using the SOAP (Subjective, Objective, Assessment, Plan) method.

**4.3 SOAP Notes—Cue Card**

Purpose: For quick reference during consultations.

**7.3 Ethics Consultation Summary Template**

Purpose: To document and communicate the key points and outcomes of an ethics consultation in a clear and balanced manner.

**4.4 Post-Consultation Survey**

Purpose: To collect standardized and quantifiable data on the effectiveness of the ethics consultation process from participants.

**4.5 Follow-Up Interview**

Purpose: To explore the nuances of participants' experiences and gather qualitative data that may not be captured through surveys. This guide is designed for semi-structured interviews, allowing for flexibility in responses while ensuring key topics are covered.

**4.6 Feedback Forms**

Purpose: To allow participants to express their thoughts and concerns freely, without fear of repercussions, especially in sensitive cases.

---

## IV. Policy Implementation and Compliance

**6.2 Ethical Risk Assessment Form**

Purpose: To identify potential ethical risks in clinical practice or organizational policies before they become critical issues.

**6.3 Incident Reporting Form for Ethical Concerns**

Purpose: To provide a mechanism for practitioners to report ethical concerns or incidents as part of an early warning system.

**6.1 Ethics Rounds Discussion Template**

Purpose: To facilitate structured and productive ethics rounds, allowing participants to explore ethical issues in a systematic way.

**6.4 Preventive Ethics Activity Log**
Purpose: To document and monitor ongoing preventive ethics activities, ensuring that they are tracked and evaluated over time.

**6.5 Ethics Audit Checklist**
Purpose: To systematically review and evaluate ethics practices within the organization as part of a preventive ethics strategy.

---

## V. Communication, Facilitation, and Training

**7.1 Active Listening and Empathetic Engagement Training Worksheet**
Purpose: To guide practitioners through exercises that enhance active listening and empathetic engagement skills.

**7.2 Mediation and Conflict Resolution Protocol**
Purpose: To provide a structured approach for mediating conflicts and facilitating consensus during ethics consultations.

**7.4 Reflective Practice and Peer Feedback Form**
Purpose: To facilitate reflection and peer feedback on communication skills following an ethics consultation.

**7.5 Communication Skills Workshop Evaluation Form**
Purpose: To evaluate the effectiveness of communication skills workshops and gather feedback for future improvement.

---

## VI. Education and Professional Development

**12.3 Continuous Education and Training Plan**
Purpose: To outline the plan for continuous education and training of ethics consultants.

**13.2 Professional Development and Continuing Education Plan**
Purpose: To outline and track participation in professional development and continuing education activities.

**13.3 Work-Life Balance Assessment Template**
Purpose: To assess and plan for balancing professional responsibilities with personal well-being.

**8.1 Training Session Planning Template**
Purpose: To guide the development of engaging and effective ethics training sessions, ensuring that all key elements are covered.

**8.3 Case Study Analysis Worksheet**
Purpose: To guide participants through the analysis of ethical case studies during training sessions.

**8.4 Simulation Scenario Template**
Purpose: To design realistic and relevant simulation scenarios for ethics training sessions, allowing participants to practice their skills in a controlled environment.

**8.2 Participant Feedback Form for Training Sessions**
Purpose: To gather structured feedback from participants on the effectiveness and relevance of the ethics training session.

**8.5 Ethics Education Program Evaluation Form**
Purpose: To evaluate the overall effectiveness of the ethics education program and gather feedback for ongoing improvement.

---

## VII. Outreach and Collaboration

**9.1 Outreach and Professional Engagement Planning Template**
Purpose: To plan and organize ethics-related education and outreach activities, ensuring that all key elements are considered.

**9.3 Networking and Collaboration Log**
Purpose: To document and track networking and collaboration efforts with other organizations, including key contacts and outcomes.

**9.5 Policy Advocacy Planning Template**
Purpose: To organize and plan bioethics-related policy advocacy efforts, ensuring that objectives and strategies are clearly defined.

**9.2 Participant Feedback Form for Outreach Events**
Purpose: To gather feedback from participants on the effectiveness and impact of the ethics-related outreach event.

**9.4 Outreach Program Evaluation Template**
Purpose: To evaluate the overall effectiveness of outreach programs and initiatives, ensuring continuous improvement.

---

## VIII. Technology, EHR, and Emerging Issues

**10.1 EHR Ethical Documentation Customization Request Form**
Purpose: To request customization of the EHR system to include specific fields and templates for ethical documentation.

**10.2 SOAP Notes**
Purpose: To ensure the effective integration of SOAP Notes into the Electronic Health Records (EHR) system, enhancing documentation practices, compliance, and patient care.

**10.3 EHR Ethical Documentation Audit Checklist**
Purpose: To ensure the accuracy, consistency, and compliance of ethical documentation within the EHR system.

**10.4 EHR Ethical Documentation Training Agenda**
Purpose: To outline the content and structure of training sessions on the use of EHR for ethical documentation.

**11.1 Digital Tools Implementation Plan**
Purpose: To outline the plan for implementing digital tools to enhance ethics rounds and training programs.

**11.2 Data Analytics Metrics and Dashboard Development Guide**
Purpose: To guide the development of metrics and dashboards for monitoring ethics consultations and training activities.

**11.3 Emerging Technology Exploration Template**
Purpose: To explore and assess new technologies for potential integration into the Bioethics Program.

## 17.1 Emerging Technologies Ethical Impact Assessment Template

Purpose: To evaluate the ethical implications of new technologies and guide decision-making within the Bioethics Program.

***

# Glossary

## A

**Abortion**
Abortion has long been a contentious issue, balancing a woman's autonomy against the rights of the fetus. In the United States, the 1973 Roe v. Wade decision established a woman's right to abortion before viability, based on privacy rights, while the 2022 Dobbs ruling left regulation to individual states. Ethical dilemmas include patient autonomy, ensuring informed consent, minimizing harm, and ensuring equitable access to abortion services. Healthcare providers must navigate moral challenges, conscientious objections, and legal complexities while prioritizing ethical standards such as autonomy, beneficence, nonmaleficence, and justice.

**Abuse**
Abuse, in its various forms—physical, emotional, sexual, and neglect—presents significant ethical and legal challenges in healthcare. Key dilemmas include balancing patient confidentiality with mandatory reporting laws, respecting patient autonomy while ensuring their safety, and navigating cultural sensitivities. Healthcare providers must prioritize autonomy, beneficence, nonmaleficence, and justice, ensuring victims receive compassionate care and protection from further harm. Mandatory reporting, legal requirements, and ethical obligations intersect in complex ways, requiring healthcare professionals to carefully balance their duties while advocating for the equitable treatment of all victims and supporting their recovery and well-being.

**Active Listening**
Active listening is a communication technique that involves fully

concentrating, understanding, responding, and remembering what the speaker is saying. It requires the listener to engage with the speaker both verbally and non-verbally, demonstrating interest through eye contact, nodding, and appropriate body language. Active listening goes beyond merely hearing words; it involves reflecting back on what is being said, asking clarifying questions, and providing feedback that shows understanding. This approach fosters trust, ensures accurate comprehension, and helps build strong relationships, making it an essential skill in healthcare, counseling, and everyday interpersonal interactions. Active listening promotes empathy, reduces misunderstandings, and supports effective problem-solving, directly aligning with patient-centered care and respecting patient autonomy.

- *Cross-reference: Patient Autonomy, Cultural Competence, Practitioner-Patient Relationship*

**Addressing Oneself and Patient**

The way healthcare providers introduce themselves and address patients is crucial for building trust and respect. Traditionally, formal introductions using titles like "Dr." maintain professional boundaries, while patient-centered care emphasizes familiarity. Key dilemmas include balancing formality and informality, respecting cultural expectations, managing power dynamics, and honoring patient preferences. Providers must be sensitive to how they address patients, respecting their autonomy while fostering trust and ensuring fairness. Legal and institutional policies influence these interactions, and ethical principles like beneficence, nonmaleficence, and justice guide the appropriate way to address patients in healthcare settings.

**Advance Directives**

Advance directives provide individuals with a legal means to express their medical treatment preferences when they can no longer communicate. These documents, including living wills and durable powers of attorney for healthcare, raise ethical challenges such as balancing patient autonomy with clinical judgment, addressing outdated directives, and resolving interpretation disputes. Surrogate decision-making and cultural considerations further complicate these situations. Healthcare providers must respect advance directives while adhering to legal requirements, institutional policies, and ethical principles like beneficence, nonmaleficence, and justice, ensuring that patient wishes align with medical standards and promote patient well-being.

- *Cross-reference: Living Will, Durable Power of Attorney (DPOA), Surrogate Decision-Making, Patient Autonomy, Informed Consent*

**Alternative Therapy**

A treatment or therapeutic approach that falls outside conventional medical practices, such as acupuncture or herbal medicine. When a patient expresses interest in an alternative therapy that diverges from medical healthcare standards of care, the practitioner should first seek to understand the patient's reasons for this interest. This allows for open communication and helps the practitioner provide informed and patient-centered care while ensuring that such therapies do not interfere with standard treatments.

**Artificial Intelligence in Healthcare**

Artificial Intelligence (AI) in healthcare refers to the use of advanced algorithms and machine learning techniques to analyze complex medical data, improve diagnostics, personalize treatment plans, and enhance patient care. AI's ability to process vast amounts of information quickly can lead to early detection of diseases, optimized treatment options, and efficient resource allocation. However, its integration raises ethical concerns about patient autonomy, privacy, and data security. Issues of algorithmic bias, accountability for AI-driven decisions, and the potential erosion of the patient-practitioner relationship must be addressed to ensure that AI applications align with the principles of beneficence, nonmaleficence, autonomy, and justice.

- *Cross-reference: Data Analytics, Patient Autonomy, Confidentiality, Ethical Decision-Making*

**Assisted Death**

Assisted death, including physician-assisted suicide (PAS) and euthanasia, raises ethical, legal, and professional dilemmas. Balancing patient autonomy with healthcare providers' ethical commitments to healing is a central issue. Ethical concerns include the potential for coercion in vulnerable populations, cultural and religious differences, and the slippery slope argument. Legal frameworks vary by state, with some allowing PAS under strict conditions. Providers must navigate these complexities while adhering to legal requirements, institutional policies, and the principles of beneficence, nonmaleficence, and justice. Providers must prioritize comprehensive palliative care and uphold ethical standards while respecting patients' end-of-life decisions.

**Autonomy**

Autonomy is the ethical principle that recognizes the right of patients to make informed, voluntary decisions about their healthcare. For autonomy to be respected, the practitioner must ensure that informed consent has been obtained, meaning that the patient or surrogate possesses the decisional capacity to understand their diagnosis, prognosis, and all available treatment options, including their associated benefits and risks. Respecting autonomy includes honoring a patient's choice even when it contradicts medical advice, provided the decision is reasonable and complies with legal and ethical standards. The decision must be made free from coercion, reflecting the patient's reasonable goals, values, and priorities while adhering to medical standards, institutional policies, and legal requirements. The final decision should be communicated clearly, documented in the medical records, and shared with all relevant healthcare team members.

- *Cross-reference: Informed Consent, Capacity, Substituted Judgment, Advance Directive*

# B

**Balance (Weigh and Balance)**

The Weigh and Balance process in ethical decision-making involves both the patient or surrogate and the practitioner collaboratively assessing the relative importance of the four primary bioethical principles: autonomy, beneficence, nonmaleficence, and justice. In the Weigh phase, they determine the weight of each principle based on the patient's reasonable goals, values, and priorities, while also considering medical standards of care, institutional policies, and legal mandates. In the Balance phase, they decide which principle or combination of principles should guide the decision-making process, aiming to arrive at a rational and reasonable recommendation that aligns with the patient's best interests and ethical obligations.

- *Cross-reference: Autonomy, Beneficence, Nonmaleficence, Justice, Ethics Consultation*

**Belmont Report**

The Belmont Report, published in 1979 by the National Commission for the Protection of Human Subjects of Biomedical and Behavioral Research, is a foundational document in the field of bioethics. It outlines ethical principles and guidelines for research involving human subjects, emphasizing respect for persons, beneficence, and justice. The report advocates for obtaining informed consent from participants, assessing risks and benefits to minimize harm, and ensuring equitable selection of subjects. These principles have shaped regulations and practices for ethical conduct in research, providing a framework to protect the rights and welfare of human subjects in biomedical and behavioral studies.

**Beneficence**

Beneficence is the ethical obligation for healthcare providers to act in the best interest of the patient, prioritizing their well-being and quality of life. To fulfill this duty, practitioners must present treatment options that align with the patient's reasonable goals, values, and priorities, ensuring that these options maximize the patient's benefits. All proposed treatments must comply with established medical standards of care, institutional policies, and legal mandates. Furthermore, the practitioner should regularly review and adjust treatment decisions to reflect any changes in the patient's condition or circumstances, ensuring that beneficence continues to guide patient care.

- *Cross-reference: Nonmaleficence, Justice, Autonomy, Weigh and Balance*

**Best Interests**

The concept of patient best interest refers to the guiding principle in healthcare decision-making that prioritizes the health, well-being, and overall welfare of the patient. Decisions are made based on what is most beneficial for the patient, considering their medical needs, personal values, and reasonable goals. This principle involves evaluating the potential benefits and burdens of treatment options, including the likelihood of achieving desired health outcomes, quality of life, and minimizing suffering. It requires healthcare providers to act with compassion, respect patient autonomy, and adhere to medical standards of care, institutional policies, and legal requirements.

**Best Practices**

Best practices are the established methods, procedures, and guidelines that are widely accepted as being the most effective and efficient ways to achieve desired outcomes in a specific field or industry. These practices are typically based on research, evidence, and expert consensus, and they serve as benchmarks for quality and performance. In healthcare, best practices aim to improve patient care, enhance safety, and optimize resource use by adhering to proven standards of clinical excellence. Organizations and professionals adopt best practices to ensure consistency, minimize risks, and maintain high standards of service, thereby promoting optimal outcomes and continuous improvement..

**Bioethics Committee**

A bioethics committee is a interprofession group that provides guidance and recommendations on ethical issues related to healthcare, medical research, and clinical practices. Comprised of healthcare professionals, ethicists, legal experts, and community representatives, these committees play a crucial role in addressing complex ethical dilemmas, such as end-of-life decisions, patient consent, allocation of scarce resources, and confidentiality. Bioethics committees review cases, develop ethical policies, and provide education and support to healthcare staff and patients. By promoting ethical standards and facilitating thoughtful deliberation, bioethics committees help ensure that patient care and medical practices align with ethical principles, legal requirements, and societal values.

**Bioethics Program Director**

A Bioethics Program Director is a leadership role responsible for overseeing and managing an institution's bioethics program. This position involves developing and implementing policies, guidelines, and educational initiatives that address ethical issues in healthcare, research, and clinical practice. The director provides expertise and guidance on complex ethical dilemmas, facilitates ethics consultations, and ensures that ethical standards align with institutional policies, medical standards of care, and legal requirements. Additionally, the Bioethics Program Director often collaborates with healthcare professionals, administrators, and ethics committees to promote ethical decision-making, enhance patient care, and uphold the institution's commitment to ethical integrity and compliance..

**Bioethics**

Bioethics is a multidisciplinary field that examines the ethical, legal, and social implications of advancements in biology, medicine, and healthcare. It addresses complex issues such as patient autonomy, informed consent, end-of-life care, reproductive rights, genetic engineering, and the allocation of scarce medical resources. Bioethics seeks to guide decision-making by applying ethical principles, such as autonomy, beneficence, nonmaleficence, and justice, to real-world dilemmas faced by patients, healthcare professionals, researchers, and policymakers. The field promotes the development of ethical guidelines, policies, and practices to ensure that biomedical and healthcare innovations are conducted in a morally responsible and socially just manner.

---

# C

### Capacity

Capacity refers to an individual's ability to understand, appreciate, and make informed decisions about their own healthcare. It involves assessing whether a person can comprehend the nature and consequences of a particular medical decision, including the benefits, risks, and alternatives. Capacity is a crucial component of informed consent and can vary depending on the complexity of the decision and the individual's cognitive and emotional state. It is not a fixed trait but can fluctuate over time and in different situations. Healthcare professionals are responsible for evaluating capacity, ensuring that patients can make autonomous and reasoned decisions about their treatment options.

- *Cross-reference: Informed Consent, Patient Autonomy, Surrogate Decision-Making, Mental Health*

### Capital Punishment

Capital punishment, or the death penalty, remains a contentious issue, raising ethical, legal, and social concerns. Ethical dilemmas include balancing justice with retribution, the risk of wrongful convictions, and whether execution methods violate the Eighth Amendment's prohibition against cruel and unusual punishment. Racial and socioeconomic disparities further complicate its fair application. Healthcare professionals face ethical conflicts when asked to participate in executions, as their role prioritizes healing, not harm. The principles of beneficence, nonmaleficence, and justice call for opposition to capital punishment and advocacy for humane treatment and fairness in the justice system.

**Case Consultation**

Case consultation is a process in healthcare ethics where a team of interdisciplinary professionals evaluates and provides guidance on complex ethical dilemmas arising in patient care. These consultations typically involve reviewing the patient's medical information, understanding the ethical issues at stake, and considering the perspectives of all involved parties, including patients, families, and healthcare providers. The goal is to reach a consensus that respects patient autonomy, adheres to ethical principles like beneficence, nonmaleficence, and justice, and complies with legal and institutional standards. Case consultations aim to support ethical decision-making, enhance patient care, and resolve conflicts in a fair and transparent manner.

**Case Studies**

Case studies are in-depth analyses of real-world or hypothetical scenarios used to explore complex issues in a specific context, often within education, healthcare, law, or business. In bioethics, case studies serve as valuable tools for examining ethical dilemmas, illustrating how ethical principles can be applied to real-life situations involving patient care and medical decision-making. By providing a detailed account of a particular situation, including background information, challenges, and possible resolutions, case studies help learners and practitioners develop critical thinking skills, understand the nuances of ethical principles, and prepare for similar situations in their professional practice.

**Chaperones**

The use of chaperones in clinical settings involves balancing patient privacy with the need for protection during sensitive examinations. While chaperones help prevent misconduct and provide reassurance, they may infringe on a patient's comfort and autonomy. Patients have the right to accept or refuse a chaperone, and healthcare providers must clearly explain their role. Cultural considerations, legal liability, and institutional policies also influence chaperone use. Ethical principles like beneficence, nonmaleficence, and justice guide the fair and respectful implementation of chaperones, ensuring patient comfort and safety while adhering to legal and institutional mandates.

**Checklists**

Checklists are structured tools used in various settings, including healthcare, to ensure that tasks are completed systematically and consistently. In clinical environments, checklists help healthcare providers follow standard protocols, enhance patient safety, and minimize errors by providing a clear, step-by-step outline of necessary actions. They serve as reminders for critical tasks, such as verifying patient identity, confirming medication dosages, or following specific procedural steps. Checklists are also used in ethical decision-making to ensure that all relevant ethical principles, legal mandates, and patient preferences are considered. Their use promotes thoroughness, accountability, and quality assurance in healthcare practices.

**Clinical Ethics Committees**

A Clinical Ethics Committee is a multidisciplinary group within a healthcare institution that provides guidance on ethical issues arising in patient care. These committees typically consist of healthcare professionals, ethicists, legal advisors, and sometimes patient representatives, working collaboratively to analyze complex ethical dilemmas, offer recommendations, and support healthcare providers and patients in making informed, ethical decisions. Clinical Ethics Committees help ensure that patient care aligns with ethical standards, institutional policies, and legal requirements by facilitating case consultations, developing ethical guidelines, and providing education and training on bioethics to healthcare staff. Their role is critical in promoting ethical integrity and patient-centered care in healthcare settings.

**Clinical Ethics Consultation**

A Clinical Ethics Consultation is a service provided by ethics experts within healthcare settings to address and resolve ethical dilemmas that arise in patient care. These consultations involve analyzing specific cases to clarify ethical issues, providing recommendations, and facilitating communication among patients, families, and healthcare teams. The goal of a clinical ethics consultation is to support informed, ethical decision-making that aligns with the patient's values, medical standards of care, and legal and institutional policies. By offering guidance on complex ethical situations, clinical ethics consultations help ensure that patient care is both ethically sound and compassionate.

**Clinical Vignettes**
Clinical vignettes are brief, descriptive scenarios that present a medical or ethical dilemma encountered in clinical practice. They are used as educational tools to facilitate learning and discussion among healthcare professionals, students, and ethics committees. By depicting realistic patient cases, clinical vignettes help illustrate complex medical conditions, ethical challenges, and decision-making processes, allowing participants to apply theoretical knowledge to practical situations. These narratives often include details about the patient's medical history, symptoms, and the ethical issues involved, encouraging critical thinking, problem-solving, and the application of ethical principles and best practices in a controlled, reflective environment..

**Confidentiality**
Confidentiality is a cornerstone of the patient-provider relationship, ensuring the privacy of personal health information (PHI). Ethical dilemmas arise when maintaining confidentiality conflicts with public safety, legal requirements, or the patient's welfare. Balancing patient privacy with obligations to disclose in situations like reporting infectious diseases or abuse is complex. Legal frameworks like HIPAA govern confidentiality practices, and unauthorized disclosures can harm patient trust. Healthcare providers must protect patient information while ensuring their actions align with ethical principles like autonomy, beneficence,

nonmaleficence, and justice, respecting patients' reasonable goals and complying with legal standards.

**Conflict of Interest**

A conflict of interest arises when a healthcare professional's personal, financial, or other secondary interests could compromise their professional judgment and commitment to the patient's best interests. Conflicts may occur in relationships with the pharmaceutical industry, clinical research, or dual administrative roles. Ethical dilemmas center on transparency, maintaining impartiality, and balancing personal interests with professional responsibilities. Healthcare providers must disclose potential conflicts to maintain patient trust, uphold autonomy, and ensure that care aligns with ethical principles like beneficence, nonmaleficence, and justice. Managing conflicts ethically preserves the integrity of patient care and complies with legal standards.

**Consent, Minors**

Consent for minors refers to the legal and ethical requirement to obtain permission from a parent or legal guardian for medical treatment or participation in research involving individuals under a certain age, typically 18 years. Because minors are generally considered not to have the full legal capacity to make informed healthcare decisions, parents or guardians must provide consent on their behalf. In some cases, minors can consent to their own treatment, especially if they are deemed "mature minors," or in situations involving reproductive health, mental health services, or treatment for substance abuse, depending on state laws and regulations.

**Continuing Education**

Continuing education refers to the ongoing professional development activities that individuals engage in to maintain, enhance, and expand their knowledge, skills, and competencies throughout their careers. In the healthcare field, continuing education is essential for keeping up-to-date with the latest medical research, technological advancements, and evolving best practices. It often involves attending workshops, conferences, courses, and seminars, as well as completing online training and certifications. By participating in continuing education, healthcare professionals can ensure they provide high-quality, evidence-based care, meet licensure requirements, and adapt to changes in their respective fields, ultimately improving patient outcomes and advancing their professional expertise.

**Contraception**

Contraception has been central to debates around reproductive rights, autonomy, and healthcare access. Ethical dilemmas arise from religious and moral opposition, disparities in access, and ensuring informed consent. Healthcare providers must balance respecting patient autonomy, providing comprehensive contraceptive options, and minimizing harm while adhering to ethical principles like beneficence, nonmaleficence, and justice. Ensuring equitable access to contraception, particularly for vulnerable populations, and navigating legal and cultural considerations are critical. Managing these complexities requires aligning care with the patient's reasonable goals, values, and priorities within the framework of medical standards and legal mandates

**CRISPR Gene Editing**

CRISPR gene editing is a revolutionary technology that enables precise alterations to DNA, offering the potential to correct genetic disorders, prevent diseases, and enhance human traits. While it holds promise for treating conditions like cystic fibrosis and sickle cell anemia, its use raises significant ethical concerns. Issues include the potential for unintended genetic changes, the long-term impacts on future generations, and the ethical implications of editing human embryos. CRISPR also poses questions about consent, accessibility, and equity in healthcare. To navigate these challenges, its application must align with ethical principles of autonomy, beneficence, nonmaleficence, and justice.

▸ *Cross-reference: Genetic Information Nondiscrimination Act (GINA), Patient Autonomy, Informed Consent, Ethical Decision-Making*

**Cultural Competence**

Cultural competence is the ability of healthcare providers and organizations to understand, respect, and effectively interact with patients from diverse cultural backgrounds. This competence involves recognizing the cultural beliefs, values, and practices that influence a patient's health behaviors and decisions. Culturally competent care requires healthcare professionals to be aware of their own cultural biases, acquire knowledge about different cultural perspectives, and develop skills to communicate and deliver care that respects patients' cultural preferences. The goal of cultural competence is to improve patient outcomes, enhance patient satisfaction, and reduce health disparities by ensuring that care is responsive to the cultural and linguistic needs of all patients.

---

# D

**Data Analytics**

Data analytics involves the systematic computational analysis of data to uncover patterns, correlations, and insights that can inform decision-making processes. In healthcare, data analytics is used to analyze patient data, clinical outcomes, operational efficiency, and other key performance indicators. By employing techniques such as statistical analysis, machine learning, and predictive modeling, healthcare professionals can identify trends, optimize treatment plans, enhance patient care, and reduce costs. Data analytics also plays a crucial role in public health for tracking disease outbreaks, improving population health management, and supporting evidence-based policy decisions. The ultimate goal is to leverage data to improve health outcomes and operational effectiveness.

**Death with Dignity — Assisted Dying**

"Death with Dignity" refers to laws allowing terminally ill patients to request life-ending medication to die on their own terms. Ethical dilemmas arise from balancing patient autonomy with moral, religious, and legal opposition, while protecting vulnerable populations from coercion. Healthcare providers must navigate complex issues such as beneficence, nonmaleficence, and justice, ensuring informed, voluntary decisions. Legal permissibility varies across states, but it does not determine professional standards. Upholding patient rights while adhering to ethical guidelines is crucial for maintaining the integrity of healthcare and public trust.

**Decision-Making Capacity**
Decision-making capacity refers to an individual's ability to understand, evaluate, and make informed decisions about their own medical care. This involves the ability to comprehend relevant information about a condition and its treatment options, appreciate the consequences of various choices, reason through the options in a logical and coherent manner, and communicate a clear and consistent choice. Assessing decision-making capacity is crucial in healthcare, especially when patients face complex medical decisions or when consent for treatment is required. A patient's capacity may be influenced by factors such as mental health conditions, cognitive impairments, or the effects of medications, and it can vary over time.

**Declaration of Geneva**
The Declaration of Geneva, adopted by the World Medical Association (WMA) in 1948, is a modern restatement of the Hippocratic Oath, outlining the ethical duties of physicians. It was created in response to the atrocities committed during World War II, emphasizing the physician's role in preserving human life and dignity. The Declaration pledges respect for human life, dedication to serving humanity, and a commitment to the principles of medical ethics, regardless of a patient’s status, race, religion, or nationality. It has been revised over time to address contemporary issues in medical ethics, such as patient autonomy, confidentiality,

and the importance of treating patients with respect and compassion.

**Deontological Ethics**

Deontological ethics is a moral theory that emphasizes the importance of following ethical principles and duties regardless of the consequences. Rooted in the works of Immanuel Kant, this approach argues that actions are morally right or wrong based on their adherence to rules, duties, or obligations rather than their outcomes. According to deontological ethics, certain actions are intrinsically right or wrong, and individuals have a moral duty to act according to these principles. This theory prioritizes the adherence to moral laws or duties, such as honesty or justice, over the pursuit of overall good or utility.

**Digital Health Ethics**

Digital health ethics encompasses the ethical considerations surrounding the use of digital technologies in healthcare, such as mobile health apps, telemedicine, wearable devices, and electronic health records. Key ethical issues include safeguarding patient privacy, ensuring data security, maintaining the integrity and accuracy of digital health information, and managing consent for data collection and use. There are also concerns about equitable access to digital health tools, potential biases in algorithms, and the impact on the patient-practitioner relationship. To address these challenges, digital health practices must adhere to ethical principles of autonomy, beneficence, nonmaleficence, and justice.

- *Cross-reference: Electronic Health Records (EHR), Patient Autonomy, Confidentiality, Telemedicine*

**Disagreement — Attending vs Resident**

Disagreements between attending physicians and residents are common in healthcare, reflecting the dynamic between experienced professionals and those in training. While attendings hold ultimate responsibility for patient care, residents contribute fresh perspectives informed by recent training. Ethical dilemmas arise when opinions diverge on diagnoses, treatment options, or patient autonomy, often complicated by the need to align with medical standards, institutional policies, and legal mandates. Balancing respect for resident input with patient-centered care requires clear communication, mutual respect, and adherence to bioethical principles like autonomy, beneficence, nonmaleficence, and justice. Managing disagreements effectively ensures patient safety and professional growth.

**Do-Not-Resuscitate Orders (DNR)**
Do-Not-Resuscitate (DNR) orders allow patients to refuse cardiopulmonary resuscitation (CPR) in situations where resuscitation may not align with their values or prognosis. These orders balance the ethical principles of autonomy, beneficence, nonmaleficence, and justice, allowing patients to make informed decisions about their end-of-life care. Ethical dilemmas often arise from the tension between respecting patient autonomy and healthcare providers' duty to preserve life. Proper documentation, clear communication, and consideration of legal and ethical guidelines are crucial to ensuring that DNR orders are respected, thus promoting patient dignity and avoiding unnecessary harm.

**Doctrine of Double Effect**
The Doctrine of Double Effect (DDE) is a moral principle asserting that an action with both good and bad effects is permissible if the intent behind the action is to achieve the good effect, with the bad effect being a foreseen but unintended consequence. Originating from Thomas Aquinas' Natural Law tradition, DDE is often invoked in healthcare to justify treatments that alleviate suffering but may hasten death. Modern bioethics challenges DDE for its focus on practitioner intention, arguing that it inadequately addresses the need for patient autonomy and informed consent, which are foundational to ethical medical practice today.

**Durable Power of Attorney (DPOA)**
A Durable Power of Attorney is a legal document that grants a

designated individual, known as the agent or attorney-in-fact, the authority to make decisions on behalf of the principal (the person granting the power) if they become incapacitated or unable to make decisions for themselves. Unlike a regular Power of Attorney, a DPOA remains effective even if the principal loses mental capacity. This document can cover a broad range of matters, including financial, legal, and healthcare decisions. In healthcare contexts, a DPOA for healthcare allows the agent to make medical decisions according to the principal's wishes, values, and best interests

---

# E

**Electronic Health Records (EHR)**
Electronic Health Records (EHR) are digital versions of patients' paper charts, encompassing comprehensive and real-time data about a patient's medical history, diagnoses, medications, treatment plans, immunization dates, allergies, radiology images, and laboratory test results. EHRs are designed to be accessed by authorized healthcare providers and staff across different healthcare settings, facilitating coordinated care and improving the quality and safety of patient care. They also support clinical decision-making by integrating evidence-based tools and guidelines. EHRs enhance communication, streamline workflows, and contribute to more accurate and efficient healthcare delivery, while also safeguarding patient privacy through secure access protocols..

**Email and Electronic Communication**
Email and electronic communication have transformed healthcare by offering speed and efficiency in patient-provider interactions. However, these methods present ethical and legal concerns, particularly regarding patient privacy, data security, and informed consent. The Health Insurance Portability and Accountability Act

(HIPAA) mandates that communications containing Protected Health Information (PHI) be HIPAA-compliant, leading many providers to use secure patient portals rather than traditional email. These portals enhance patient privacy, ensure legal compliance, and maintain accountability. While electronic communication improves accessibility, healthcare providers must balance the benefits with the need to protect patient information and uphold ethical standards like autonomy and nonmaleficence.

**Emergency Medical Treatment and Labor Act (EMTALA)**
The Emergency Medical Treatment and Labor Act (EMTALA) is a federal law enacted in 1986 that requires hospitals with emergency departments to provide emergency medical care to anyone needing treatment, regardless of their insurance status, ability to pay, or citizenship. Under EMTALA, hospitals must conduct a medical screening to determine if an emergency medical condition exists and provide stabilizing treatment if necessary. If a hospital is unable to stabilize a patient, it must arrange for a proper transfer to another facility that can provide the necessary care. EMTALA is a critical safeguard to ensure access to emergency medical services and prevent patient dumping.

**Errors**
Errors in healthcare pose ethical and legal concerns, impacting patient safety, provider integrity, and trust in the healthcare system. Key dilemmas include transparency, disclosure, and accountability. Historically, providers feared litigation or damage to reputation from disclosing errors, but modern ethical standards demand openness to respect patient autonomy. Failure to disclose errors violates patients' rights, undermines informed consent, and may result in legal consequences. Ethical principles such as beneficence, nonmaleficence, and justice require that errors be disclosed to prevent harm, improve patient safety, and ensure fair treatment for all. Transparency fosters trust and supports ethical, patient-centered care.

**Ethics Consultant**

An ethics consultant is a professional who provides expertise in ethical decision-making within healthcare settings. Their role involves offering guidance on complex ethical issues, helping to resolve conflicts, and ensuring that patient care aligns with ethical principles such as autonomy, beneficence, nonmaleficence, and justice. Ethics consultants work closely with patients, families, and healthcare teams to facilitate communication, clarify ethical dilemmas, and recommend ethically appropriate actions. They may also contribute to policy development, education, and training within their institutions. Ethics consultants are vital in promoting ethical standards and enhancing the quality of care in healthcare organizations..

**Ethics Consultation**

Ethics consultation is a process through which healthcare professionals, patients, or their families seek guidance on complex ethical issues that arise in clinical practice. The purpose of ethics consultation is to support informed and ethical decision-making, ensuring that patient care aligns with ethical principles such as autonomy, beneficence, nonmaleficence, and justice. During an ethics consultation, an ethics consultant or ethics committee reviews the case, engages with the relevant stakeholders, and provides recommendations to help resolve ethical dilemmas. These consultations play a crucial role in addressing conflicts, clarifying values, and promoting ethically sound practices in healthcare settings.

**Ethics Rounds**

Ethics rounds are structured discussions held within healthcare settings where a multidisciplinary team of healthcare professionals, including physicians, nurses, social workers, and ethics consultants, gather to review and analyze ethical issues related to patient care. These rounds provide a forum for team members to discuss challenging cases, reflect on ethical dilemmas, and explore the application of ethical principles such as autonomy, beneficence, nonmaleficence, and justice. Ethics rounds contribute to the ongoing education of healthcare providers, promote an ethical culture within healthcare organizations, and support ethical decision-making by integrating ethical considerations into clinical practice.

- *Cross-reference: Ethics Consultation, Clinical Ethics Committees, Case Consultation*

**Euthanasia**

Euthanasia, the intentional ending of a person's life by a healthcare professional to alleviate suffering, raises significant ethical, legal, and philosophical challenges. The practice is illegal in the United States, where end-of-life care focuses on alternatives like palliative care. Key ethical dilemmas include balancing patient autonomy, the sanctity of life, and the physician's duty to do no harm. While some argue for euthanasia as an act of compassion, professional guidelines reject it, emphasizing patient care through legally and ethically accepted means like pain management and hospice. The debate centers on respecting life, patient rights, and ethical boundaries.

---

# F

**Financial Disclosures**

Financial disclosures in healthcare involve the transparent reporting of financial relationships between healthcare providers and external entities, such as pharmaceutical companies or medical device manufacturers. These disclosures are essential to avoiding conflicts of interest, ensuring patient trust, and maintaining the integrity of clinical decision-making. The Physician Payments Sunshine Act mandates transparency in these relationships, aiming to prevent undue influence on patient care. Ethical guidelines from organizations like the AMA emphasize the need for financial transparency to protect patient welfare, uphold autonomy, and ensure that medical decisions are free from bias.

**Four Principles — Principlism**
This foundational framework of biomedical ethics guides ethical decision-making by emphasizing four key principles. Patient Autonomy (Informed Consent): This principle respects the rights of patients to make informed decisions about their own healthcare based on their goals, values, and priorities. Practitioner Beneficence (Maximize Benefits): It focuses on acting in the patient's best interests to promote their well-being and enhance their quality of life. Practitioner Nonmaleficence (Minimize Burdens): This principle is about avoiding harm and minimizing the burdens of treatment on the patient. Public Justice (Ensure Fairness): It ensures that fairness and equity are upheld in the distribution of healthcare resources and treatment options.

**Futile Treatment**
Futile treatment refers to medical interventions that are unlikely to benefit the patient, particularly in end-of-life situations. This concept raises ethical dilemmas regarding patient autonomy, healthcare providers' professional judgment, and the allocation of resources. While patients or families may request continued treatment, healthcare professionals must balance these requests with the ethical duty to avoid administering ineffective care. Futile treatment often involves conflicts over the definition of "benefit" and requires clear communication to align care with the patient's reasonable goals, values, and priorities, while upholding ethical principles such as beneficence, nonmaleficence, and justice.

---

# G

**Genetic Information Nondiscrimination Act (GINA)**
The Genetic Information Nondiscrimination Act (GINA) of 2008 prohibits the misuse of genetic information in health insurance and employment. It protects individuals from discrimination based on genetic predispositions to certain diseases. GINA ensures that

genetic data cannot be used by employers or insurers to make decisions about hiring, coverage, or premiums. By safeguarding privacy and promoting fairness, GINA supports patient autonomy and encourages genetic testing without fear of negative repercussions, fostering public trust in personalized medicine. This legislation aligns with the ethical principles of nonmaleficence, beneficence, justice, and respect for patient autonomy.

**Gift Acceptance**
Gift acceptance in healthcare involves ethical considerations surrounding the influence of gifts on medical judgment and patient care. While gifts were historically seen as expressions of gratitude, contemporary concerns focus on the potential for gifts from patients or commercial entities to affect clinical decisions. Accepting gifts may blur professional boundaries and create conflicts of interest, undermining trust and patient autonomy. Ethical guidelines, such as those from the AMA, advise against accepting gifts that could influence decision-making, prioritizing transparency, fairness, and the patient's best interests to maintain professional integrity and uphold ethical standards in patient care.

**Gunshot Wounds and Mandatory Reporting**
Gunshot wounds (GSWs) present ethical and legal challenges for healthcare providers, particularly due to mandatory reporting laws that require disclosing GSW incidents to law enforcement. These laws aim to protect public safety but can conflict with patient privacy and autonomy. Healthcare providers must balance their duty to report with ethical obligations to maintain confidentiality, minimize harm, and ensure justice. Reporting only the minimum required information and being transparent with patients about these legal requirements helps to maintain trust while adhering to public safety regulations, aligning with the ethical principles of autonomy, beneficence, nonmaleficence, and justice.

# H

**Health Insurance Portability and Accountability Act (HIPAA)**
The Health Insurance Portability and Accountability Act (HIPAA) is a U.S. federal law enacted in 1996 that aims to protect the privacy and security of individuals' medical information. HIPAA establishes national standards for the handling, storage, and transmission of protected health information (PHI), ensuring that patient data remains confidential and secure. The law also grants patients rights over their health information, including the right to access their medical records and request corrections. Additionally, HIPAA includes provisions that facilitate the portability of health insurance coverage for individuals transitioning between jobs, thereby protecting health coverage continuity

**Healthcare Standards of Care**
Standard of care refers to the level and quality of care that a reasonably competent healthcare professional, with a similar background and in a similar community, would provide under comparable circumstances. It serves as a benchmark for assessing the appropriateness and effectiveness of medical treatment and interventions. The standard of care is determined by various factors, including clinical guidelines, expert opinions, medical literature, and prevailing practices. Adherence to the standard of care ensures that patients receive safe and effective treatment, while deviations from this standard may lead to medical liability or malpractice claims if harm results

**Hippocratic Oath**
The Hippocratic Oath is a seminal ethical code of conduct historically attributed to the ancient Greek physician Hippocrates and serves as a foundational text for medical ethics. Traditionally taken by physicians, the Oath commits them to practicing medicine ethically and honestly, emphasizing principles such as patient confidentiality, nonmaleficence "*do no harm*" and beneficence

(acting in the patient's best interests). It includes commitments to avoid causing harm or injustice, refraining from exploiting patients, and upholding professional integrity. While the Oath has evolved over centuries, its core tenets continue to influence contemporary medical ethics and guide healthcare professionals in their practice.

**Hospice Care**

Hospice care provides comfort and support for patients with terminal illnesses, focusing on improving quality of life rather than curing illness. It involves symptom management, emotional support, and addressing the spiritual needs of patients and their families. Ethical dilemmas arise in balancing the transition from curative to palliative care, respecting patient autonomy, and ensuring equitable access to services. Hospice care emphasizes beneficence (maximizing patient comfort), nonmaleficence (avoiding harm from unnecessary treatments), autonomy (informed decision-making), and justice (fair access to care), ensuring that patient care aligns with ethical and legal standards.

---

## I

**Immunization — Vaccine Hesitancy**

Vaccine hesitancy refers to the reluctance or refusal to vaccinate despite the availability of vaccines, a challenge that affects public health, especially when healthcare providers exhibit hesitancy. Historical resistance to vaccines has evolved into contemporary concerns about safety, efficacy, and ethical issues. Among healthcare practitioners, vaccine hesitancy undermines public trust and patient safety. Ethical dilemmas arise when personal beliefs conflict with professional duties to promote health and prevent harm. Healthcare providers are ethically obligated to prioritize beneficence, nonmaleficence, and justice by advocating for immunization to protect patients and the broader community.

**Impaired Drivers and Reporting**

Reporting impaired drivers involves legal and ethical responsibilities for healthcare practitioners to ensure public safety while balancing patient confidentiality. Impairment can result from alcohol, medications, or medical conditions like epilepsy and dementia. Healthcare providers face ethical dilemmas between respecting patient autonomy and protecting public safety. Legal requirements for reporting impaired drivers vary by jurisdiction, and mandatory reporting may strain the patient-provider relationship. Practitioners must prioritize beneficence and nonmaleficence by preventing harm, ensuring fair application of reporting laws (justice), and maintaining clear communication with patients about the potential consequences of their health conditions on driving abilities.

**Impaired Practitioners — Reporting**

Reporting impaired practitioners is a crucial responsibility in healthcare, balancing patient safety with the rights and privacy of healthcare workers. Historically, the stigma around addiction or mental health issues in healthcare created silence around reporting. Today, healthcare practitioners face ethical dilemmas, such as the conflict between loyalty to colleagues and the duty to protect patients. Legal obligations vary by jurisdiction, but reporting is often mandated to prevent harm. Ethical principles like nonmaleficence and justice guide the need to ensure impaired practitioners receive help while prioritizing patient safety and maintaining public trust in the healthcare system.

**Informed Consent**

Informed consent is a fundamental ethical and legal requirement in healthcare, ensuring that patients or their surrogates have the ability to make voluntary and informed decisions about their medical care. For informed consent to be valid, several conditions must be met: the patient or surrogate must have decisional capacity to understand and make choices about their care; they must be fully informed of their diagnosis and prognosis, available treatment options (including no treatment), and the benefits and risks associated with each option. The decision must be made without coercion, aligning with the patient's reasonable goals, values, and priorities. Finally, the decision must be communicated, documented in medical records, and shared with all relevant healthcare team members to ensure cohesive and ethical care

**Interrogation — Healthcare Boundaries**
Healthcare professionals' involvement in interrogations has been historically contentious, particularly regarding ethical standards in wartime and conflict. The Nuremberg Code, developed after World War II, set clear ethical guidelines prohibiting healthcare professionals from participating in coercive interrogations, which often involve physical or psychological harm. Contemporary dilemmas include balancing legal pressures with ethical duties to "do no harm." Professionals must uphold patient autonomy, beneficence, nonmaleficence, and justice, avoiding complicity in practices that violate human rights and undermine medical ethics. Their role is to heal, not to harm, ensuring that care and respect for individuals remain paramount.

- *Cross-reference: Autonomy, Capacity, Surrogate Decision-Making, Youth Consent*

---

# J

**Justice**
Justice refers to the ethical obligation of healthcare practitioners to ensure fairness in the delivery of care. To implement justice as fairness, practitioners must provide treatment options that are equitable, ensuring that all patients receive appropriate care based on their medical needs, without discrimination or bias. These options must adhere to medical standards of care, institutional policies, and legal mandates, ensuring that all patients are treated with respect and dignity. By upholding the principle of public

justice, practitioners contribute to a healthcare system that is fair, just, and committed to the equal treatment of all individuals.

- *Cross-reference: Autonomy, Beneficence, Nonmaleficence, Structural Injustice in Healthcare, Resource Allocation*

---

# K

### Kantian Ethics

Kantian ethics, rooted in the philosophy of Immanuel Kant, is a deontological ethical theory that prioritizes the inherent morality of actions based on adherence to duty and universal moral laws. According to Kantian principles, actions are morally right if they conform to a universal maxim that can be consistently willed as a universal law. In medical ethics, this approach emphasizes the respect for patient autonomy, requiring healthcare professionals to act with honesty and respect, treating patients as ends in themselves rather than means to an end. Kantian ethics stresses that moral actions are determined by duty and the intrinsic worth of individuals, regardless of the consequences.

---

# L

### Lifelong Learning

Lifelong learning is the continuous process of acquiring and updating medical knowledge and skills throughout a healthcare professional's career. Historically, medical education evolved from apprenticeships to formalized, structured learning, underscoring the need for ongoing education. Today, lifelong learning is essential for staying current with advancements in medical science, technology, and evidence-based practices. It ensures that healthcare providers meet professional, legal, and ethical standards, aligning with the principles of beneficence, nonmaleficence, and patient autonomy. By engaging in continuing education, practitioners can provide informed, high-quality care, ensuring that patient outcomes improve and healthcare standards are consistently maintained.

**Living Will**

A living will is a legal document that allows individuals to specify their preferences for medical treatment and end-of-life care in advance, in the event that they become incapacitated or unable to communicate their wishes. It typically outlines instructions regarding life-sustaining measures, such as the use of ventilators, feeding tubes, resuscitation efforts, and other interventions. By providing clear directives, a living will helps ensure that healthcare decisions align with the individual's values, beliefs, and desires, reducing uncertainty for family members and healthcare providers. It is an essential component of advance care planning, promoting patient autonomy and informed decision-making.

- *Cross-reference: Advance Directive, Durable Power of Attorney (DPOA), Patient Autonomy, End-of-Life Care*

---

# M

**Malpractice — Medical**

Medical malpractice refers to a healthcare professional's failure to meet the accepted standard of care, resulting in harm to a patient. This concept dates back to ancient civilizations, with modern definitions shaped by legal and ethical guidelines. Key elements of malpractice include duty, breach of duty, causation, and damages. Malpractice cases arise from failures in communication, inadequate informed consent, or medical negligence. Ethical principles such as beneficence, nonmaleficence, and justice guide practitioners in avoiding malpractice by ensuring they act in the patient's best interest, minimize harm, and provide care that aligns with professional standards and patient rights.

**Media Communications**

Media communications in healthcare have historically been vital for public health campaigns, from early 20th-century efforts combating diseases like polio to modern digital health updates. While media enables widespread dissemination of information, ethical dilemmas arise regarding accuracy, potential public panic, and the balance between transparency and confidentiality. In today's digital age, misinformation can rapidly affect public trust and health behaviors, highlighting the need for responsible, evidence-based communication. Healthcare providers must adhere to ethical principles of autonomy, beneficence, and nonmaleficence, ensuring patient privacy is respected while providing clear, beneficial, and harm-free public health information.

**Mediation**

Mediation is a structured, voluntary process in which a neutral third party, known as the mediator, facilitates communication and negotiation between disputing parties to help them reach a mutually acceptable resolution. Unlike arbitration or litigation, mediation does not involve imposing a decision; instead, the mediator assists the parties in exploring their interests, identifying common ground, and developing solutions that satisfy both sides. Mediation is commonly used in various settings, including healthcare, family disputes, workplace conflicts, and legal cases, to resolve conflicts efficiently and amicably while preserving relationships and allowing parties to maintain control over the outcome.

**Medical Records**

Medical records are vital documents that track a patient's health history and treatments. Historically, they were controlled solely by healthcare providers, but evolving patient rights movements, particularly with the Health Insurance Portability and Accountability Act (HIPAA) in 1996, have shifted focus to patient autonomy. HIPAA ensures patients' right to access and control their

Protected Health Information (PHI) while maintaining strict confidentiality. While Electronic Health Records (EHRs) enhance accessibility, they also raise concerns about privacy breaches. Balancing easy access to medical records with stringent privacy measures is crucial for upholding legal and ethical responsibilities in healthcare.

**Minor Patients**
Minor patients present unique ethical and legal challenges in healthcare. Historically, healthcare decisions were made by parents or guardians under the principle of *parens patriae*, with limited consideration of minors' autonomy. Over time, particularly in cases involving reproductive health and mental health care, minors' rights have expanded. Contemporary dilemmas involve balancing minors' autonomy with parental authority and legal mandates. While state laws vary, many allow minors to consent to certain types of care. Healthcare providers must respect minors' emerging autonomy, involve them in decision-making, and ensure care aligns with legal and ethical standards to prioritize their best interests.

---

# N

**Nonmaleficence**
Nonmaleficence is the ethical principle requiring healthcare providers to avoid causing harm and to minimize the burdens on the patient. To uphold nonmaleficence, practitioners must offer treatment options that reduce potential physical, emotional, or psychological burdens, ensuring that these align with the patient's reasonable goals, values, and priorities. All treatment options presented must adhere to established medical standards of care, institutional policies, and legal mandates. By carefully selecting and managing treatment approaches, practitioners can prevent unnecessary suffering and safeguard the patient's well-being, consistently maintaining the commitment to do no harm.

- *Cross-reference: Beneficence, Justice, Autonomy, Weigh and Balance, Medical Harm*

**Nurses and Allied Health Professionals**

Nurses and allied health professionals have historically been viewed as supporting roles within a physician-led healthcare system. Over time, their roles have expanded, with many taking on greater decision-making responsibilities and providing direct patient care. Today, professionals such as nurse practitioners, physician assistants, and physical therapists are key to managing chronic conditions, preventive care, and patient education. This shift presents challenges related to scope of practice, interprofessional collaboration, and professional autonomy. These healthcare providers must navigate complex ethical, legal, and institutional frameworks to ensure patient care aligns with beneficence, nonmaleficence, autonomy, and justice.

---

# O

**Organ Donations**

Organ donation has evolved significantly since the first successful transplant in 1954, transforming from a rare procedure to a vital part of modern healthcare. Ethical concerns include informed consent, the allocation of scarce organs, and the determination of death. Contemporary dilemmas involve balancing donor autonomy with public health needs, addressing disparities in organ availability, and ensuring fair access to transplants. Federal laws such as the National Organ Transplant Act (NOTA) and the Uniform Anatomical Gift Act (UAGA) provide legal frameworks to safeguard donors and recipients. Ethical considerations focus on maximizing benefits while minimizing harm and ensuring justice in the distribution of organs.

**Organizational Ethics**

Organizational ethics refers to the principles, values, and standards that guide the behavior and decision-making processes within an organization. It encompasses the moral responsibilities of the organization toward its stakeholders, including employees, customers, suppliers, and the broader community. Organizational ethics involves establishing codes of conduct, ethical guidelines, and policies that promote integrity, accountability, fairness, and transparency. It also includes the creation of ethical cultures and frameworks to address ethical dilemmas, compliance with laws and regulations, and the promotion of ethical leadership. The goal is to ensure that all organizational activities align with ethical principles and contribute positively to society.

---

# P

**Palliative Care**

Palliative care focuses on relieving suffering and improving the quality of life for patients with serious illnesses, integrating medical care with emotional, social, and spiritual support. Historically, healthcare emphasized life-prolonging treatments, often compromising patient comfort. The hospice movement led to the development of palliative care, advocating for a patient-centered approach that honors individual goals and values. Contemporary dilemmas include the timing of palliative care introduction, misconceptions about its role, and disparities in access. Legal frameworks such as the Patient Self-Determination Act (PSDA) ensure patient autonomy, while ethical principles emphasize maximizing benefits, minimizing harm, and ensuring equitable care for all patients.

**Patient-Practitioner Relationship**

The patient-practitioner relationship has shifted from a historically paternalistic approach, where practitioners made decisions without patient input, to a more collaborative model emphasizing patient autonomy. This shift, driven by the rise of patient-centered care, prioritizes shared decision-making, ensuring that care aligns with the patient's reasonable goals, values, and priorities. Ethical challenges arise in balancing practitioner expertise with patient autonomy, particularly with advancements in digital health and telemedicine. Ensuring trust, clear communication, and respect for patient rights remains critical. Legal frameworks, such as informed consent laws, support this relationship by safeguarding patient autonomy while ensuring practitioners act beneficently and minimize harm.

**Practitioner Disagreements**
Practitioner disagreements arise from differences in medical judgment, training, or interpretations of evidence-based practices. Historically, these were often resolved hierarchically, with senior practitioners making the final decisions. Modern interdisciplinary care, however, emphasizes collaborative resolution, respecting patient autonomy and promoting patient-centered outcomes. Unresolved disagreements can lead to confusion, delayed care, and potential harm, violating the principle of nonmaleficence. To resolve conflicts effectively, practitioners must balance ethical principles: autonomy (informed consent), beneficence (acting in the patient's best interest), nonmaleficence (avoiding harm), and justice (ensuring fairness in care). Structured conflict resolution processes help ensure optimal patient outcomes.

**Precision Medicine**
Precision medicine involves tailoring medical treatment to individual patient characteristics, such as genetic makeup, lifestyle, and environment. Unlike the traditional one-size-fits-all approach, it seeks to optimize patient care by personalizing therapies. While this innovative practice enhances Practitioner Beneficence by maximizing patient benefits, it also raises ethical concerns. These include Patient Autonomy (ensuring informed consent, especially regarding genetic testing implications), Practitioner Nonmaleficence (minimizing harm through responsible data use), and Public Justice (ensuring equitable access to precision medicine across diverse populations). Precision medicine offers great

potential, but practitioners must balance its benefits with ethical obligations to ensure fair, individualized care.

**Pregnant Patients**
The treatment of pregnant patients historically prioritized paternalistic decision-making, often neglecting Patient Autonomy. Contemporary practice focuses on respecting pregnant patients' rights to make informed decisions about their healthcare, balancing maternal and fetal well-being. Ethical dilemmas arise when maternal and fetal interests conflict, with principles like Practitioner Beneficence and Nonmaleficence guiding care decisions. Legal frameworks, such as the Pregnancy Discrimination Act, protect pregnant patients from unfair treatment, ensuring equitable access to care under Public Justice. Healthcare providers must respect autonomy, provide patient-centered care, minimize harm, and ensure fairness in treating both the mother and fetus.

**Preventive Ethics**
Preventive ethics refers to proactive measures and strategies designed to identify, address, and mitigate potential ethical issues before they arise in healthcare and other professional settings. This approach focuses on preventing ethical dilemmas by implementing policies, training programs, and frameworks that guide decision-making and practice. Preventive ethics involves educating professionals about ethical principles, fostering a culture of ethical awareness, and establishing procedures for early intervention and resolution of ethical concerns. By addressing potential issues in advance, preventive ethics aims to enhance the quality of carc, uphold ethical standards, and reduce the risk of ethical violations..

**Product Sales in Healthcare**
The sale of products to patients by healthcare providers raises ethical concerns related to conflicts of interest and patient trust. Historically, medical ethics emphasized a fiduciary duty, where physicians prioritized patient welfare over profit, and the introduction of direct sales risked undermining this principle.

Modern challenges include balancing Patient Autonomy by ensuring informed consent, while also adhering to Practitioner Beneficence, ensuring products benefit patients without compromising care. Legal frameworks like the Anti-Kickback Statute protect against financial exploitation. Providers must prioritize transparency and fairness (Public Justice) to avoid exploiting vulnerable populations, ensuring ethical, patient-centered care.

**Protected Health Information (PHI)**
Protected Health Information (PHI) refers to any information about an individual's health status, provision of healthcare, or payment for healthcare that can be used to identify the individual and is protected under privacy laws. PHI includes personal details such as names, addresses, dates of birth, Social Security numbers, medical records, and other health-related information. In the United States, PHI is safeguarded by the Health Insurance Portability and Accountability Act (HIPAA), which establishes standards for privacy and security to ensure that individuals' health information is kept confidential and secure from unauthorized access or disclosure.

**Public Health Ethics**
Public health ethics involves the moral considerations and principles guiding efforts to protect and promote the health of populations. Unlike clinical ethics, which focuses on individual patient care, public health ethics balances individual rights with collective well-being. Key ethical issues include ensuring fair access to healthcare resources, respecting autonomy while implementing public health measures (such as vaccination mandates and quarantine), and addressing health disparities. Public health initiatives must navigate the ethical tension between protecting individual freedoms and ensuring the common good, adhering to principles of justice, beneficence, nonmaleficence, and respect for autonomy.

▸ *Cross-reference: Justice, Autonomy, Vaccine Hesitancy, Confidentiality, Resource Allocation*

---

# Q

**Quality Improvement**

Quality improvement (QI) is a systematic approach to enhancing the effectiveness, efficiency, and safety of healthcare services and processes. It involves continuous evaluation and refinement of practices based on data-driven analysis to achieve better patient outcomes and overall organizational performance. QI initiatives typically include setting specific goals, measuring performance against benchmarks, identifying areas for improvement, and implementing evidence-based changes. The process often involves multidisciplinary teams, feedback mechanisms, and iterative testing of interventions to ensure that improvements are sustainable and aligned with best practices and patient needs. By fostering a culture of continuous improvement, QI aims to enhance healthcare delivery and patient satisfaction.

---

# R

**Racial Concordance in Healthcare**

Racial concordance refers to the practice of matching healthcare providers and patients based on race. Historically, it has been explored as a way to address racial disparities and improve patient satisfaction, particularly among minority populations. While racial concordance can foster better communication and trust, it does not necessarily guarantee higher-quality care. The ethical dilemma involves balancing patient autonomy—allowing patients to express racial preferences—with principles of justice and beneficence, ensuring all patients receive equitable, competent care. Ultimately, the goal is to build a healthcare system where racial concordance is unnecessary because all patients receive unbiased, high-quality care.

**Referral and Fee Splitting in Healthcare**
Referral and fee-splitting in healthcare, where providers receive compensation for referring patients, have raised ethical concerns historically and remain legally regulated. Fee-splitting can create conflicts of interest, compromising patient care and violating the principles of beneficence and nonmaleficence. Federal laws like the Stark Law and Anti-Kickback Statute prohibit such practices to protect patient autonomy and ensure referrals are based on clinical need, not financial gain. Ethically, providers must prioritize patient welfare, ensuring transparency in referrals and avoiding financial incentives that could undermine trust or create inequities in access to care.

**Reportable Infections and Illnesses**
Reportable infections and illnesses refer to certain diseases that healthcare providers must report to public health authorities to prevent and control outbreaks. Historically, this practice began with diseases like tuberculosis and cholera, but today it includes conditions like COVID-19, HIV, and measles. While essential for public safety, reporting can raise ethical tensions between protecting patient autonomy (privacy and consent) and fulfilling the duty of public justice (ensuring community health). Legal frameworks such as HIPAA provide exceptions for public health reporting, aiming to balance individual rights with the broader goal of beneficence and harm reduction in society.

**Research and Clinical Equipoise**
Clinical equipoise is the ethical principle that justifies conducting randomized controlled trials (RCTs) by ensuring there is genuine uncertainty in the medical community about which treatment is superior. Historically, it has safeguarded patient welfare by preventing the administration of knowingly inferior treatments. This concept aligns with the ethical principles of nonmaleficence

—ensuring no harm is done—and beneficence—aiming to maximize patient benefits. However, equipoise presents dilemmas when emerging evidence suggests one treatment's superiority, challenging researchers to uphold fairness (justice) and patient autonomy while ensuring that participants receive the best possible care based on evolving knowledge.

**Research on Human Subjects**

Research on human subjects involves ethical and legal considerations aimed at protecting participants' rights and welfare. Historical abuses, such as the Tuskegee Syphilis Study, led to the creation of key ethical guidelines, including the Nuremberg Code and the Belmont Report, which prioritize informed consent, beneficence, and justice. Federal regulations like the Common Rule mandate Institutional Review Board (IRB) oversight to ensure participant protection. The ethical challenge lies in balancing scientific progress with safeguarding individuals, ensuring that vulnerable populations are not exploited, and that research risks are minimized while potential benefits are maximized.

**Resource Allocation**

Resource allocation in healthcare refers to the ethical distribution of limited medical resources, such as organs, vaccines, or critical care beds, especially in times of scarcity. Ethical dilemmas arise in determining who should receive treatment first, balancing fairness, need, and the potential for benefit. Approaches to resource allocation often incorporate principles like justice (equitable access), beneficence (maximizing overall good), and nonmaleficence (minimizing harm). Decisions must consider both individual patient needs and the greater public health impact, ensuring transparency and fairness while avoiding discrimination and bias in the allocation process.

- *Cross-reference: Justice, Beneficence, Public Health Ethics, Triage Decision-Making, Ethical Decision-Making*

**Root Cause Analysis (RCA)**:
Root Cause Analysis is a systematic process for identifying the underlying cause of adverse events in healthcare. In the context of biomedical ethics, it upholds the four principles: 1) Autonomy by ensuring patients' perspectives are considered; 2) Beneficence by promoting better outcomes through improved systems; 3) Nonmaleficence by minimizing harm by addressing root issues; and 4) Justice by ensuring equitable access to safer care. RCA helps healthcare teams improve patient safety and quality by addressing system flaws rather than blaming individuals.

---

# S

**Self, Family, and Friends Treatment**
Treating oneself, family members, or friends presents significant ethical dilemmas due to the risk of compromised objectivity, confidentiality breaches, and conflicts of interest. Personal ties can cloud a physician's judgment, jeopardizing professional detachment needed to provide unbiased care. Ethical guidelines, such as those from the AMA, discourage this practice, emphasizing the potential harm to patient autonomy, beneficence, nonmaleficence, and public justice. Patients may withhold sensitive information, and physicians may avoid necessary procedures, resulting in suboptimal care. To ensure fairness and uphold ethical standards, physicians are advised to avoid treating individuals with whom they share personal relationships.

**Sexual Boundaries**
Sexual relationships between healthcare practitioners and patients undermine professional ethics due to the inherent power imbalance and potential for exploitation. These relationships violate patient autonomy by compromising the patient's ability to make free and informed decisions, while also undermining practitioner beneficence, as emotional involvement skews clinical judgment.

Nonmaleficence is breached when personal relationships result in emotional harm or disrupted care, and justice is denied as personal biases lead to unequal treatment. Ethical guidelines from the AMA and ACP emphasize maintaining strict professional boundaries to protect patient welfare and ensure unbiased, equitable care.

**Sexually Transmitted Infections (STIs)**
Sexually transmitted infections (STIs) refer to infections transmitted through sexual contact, which may or may not present symptoms. Historically stigmatized, STIs are now addressed through public health measures like mandatory reporting and expedited partner therapy (EPT), designed to control their spread. These interventions raise ethical dilemmas by balancing patient autonomy, confidentiality, and public health. The term STI, preferred over sexually transmitted disease (STD), reduces stigma and reflects that many infections do not progress to symptomatic disease. Managing STIs requires navigating legal, ethical, and medical responsibilities to protect both individual rights and community health.

**SOAP Notes**
The SOAP Notes Template provides a structured approach for documenting ethics consultations in healthcare, focusing on the bioethical principles of autonomy, beneficence, nonmaleficence, and justice. It includes four sections: Subjective, capturing the patient's or surrogate's perspective on their medical condition, diagnosis, prognosis, and treatment options, including ethical considerations; Objective, recording clinical facts and ensuring they align with medical standards of care; Assessment, evaluating the ethical issues, summarizing the THINK and ASSESS steps, and applying the TAC analysis to each bioethical principle; and Plan, outlining the recommended course of action, communication strategies, and adherence to ethical, legal, and medical standards.

**Social Media Boundaries in Healthcare**
Social media in healthcare presents unique ethical challenges, requiring healthcare professionals to balance personal expression

with patient confidentiality and professional integrity. Historically, healthcare interactions were confined to private consultations, but social media blurs these boundaries. Key dilemmas involve protecting patient privacy under laws like HIPAA, avoiding the disclosure of identifiable health information, and maintaining professional distance. Healthcare providers must ensure that their online presence adheres to ethical guidelines, such as those outlined by the AMA, to protect patient trust, confidentiality, and fairness, while responsibly using social media to promote public health.

**Stages of Grief**
The stages of grief, introduced by psychiatrist Elisabeth Kübler-Ross, outline the emotional responses individuals may experience when coping with significant loss or change. These stages include denial (initial shock and disbelief), anger (frustration and resentment), bargaining (attempts to reverse or mitigate the loss), depression (deep sadness and withdrawal), and acceptance (coming to terms with the loss and finding a way to move forward). While not necessarily experienced sequentially or by everyone, this model provides a framework for understanding the complex and personal process of grieving, recognizing that each individual's experience is unique.

**Sterilization in Healthcare**
Sterilization in healthcare, a permanent method of contraception, presents significant ethical concerns due to its historical misuse and the complexity of ensuring informed consent. Historically, involuntary sterilizations were performed on marginalized populations, leading to human rights violations. Today, sterilization must be voluntary, with a focus on protecting patient autonomy and preventing coercion. Ethical dilemmas persist around ensuring that patients fully understand the procedure’s consequences, particularly for vulnerable groups. Balancing patient rights, informed consent, and equitable access to sterilization is essential

for upholding the principles of autonomy, beneficence, nonmaleficence, and justice.

**Strikes and Unionization in Healthcare**
Strikes and unionization in healthcare present ethical dilemmas, as they balance healthcare workers' rights with the duty to ensure patient care. Historically, healthcare unions have advocated for better working conditions and patient care standards. However, strikes raise concerns about disrupting essential services, impacting patient well-being. Ethical challenges revolve around upholding patient autonomy, minimizing harm (nonmaleficence), promoting patient welfare (beneficence), and ensuring fairness (justice). While labor laws protect workers' rights to unionize, healthcare professionals must carefully manage strikes to ensure patients receive necessary care, adhering to bioethical principles to maintain patient trust and public health.

**Structural Injustice in Healthcare**
Structural injustice in healthcare refers to the systemic inequalities that lead to disparities in access, treatment, and outcomes for marginalized populations. Historically rooted in discriminatory practices such as racial segregation and biases in medical care, these injustices persist in modern healthcare. Examples include the Tuskegee Syphilis Study and ongoing disparities in maternal mortality among African American women. Addressing structural injustice requires healthcare providers to ensure equitable access, culturally competent care, and the dismantling of systemic barriers that perpetuate inequality. Ethical principles such as autonomy, beneficence, nonmaleficence, and justice guide efforts to rectify these long-standing inequities.

**Student Involvement in Patient Care**
Student involvement in patient care is a crucial component of medical education, offering students hands-on clinical experience under supervision. However, this practice raises ethical concerns, particularly regarding patient autonomy and informed consent.

Patients must be fully informed about the role of students in their care and provide explicit consent. Ethical principles like beneficence and nonmaleficence require careful supervision to ensure patient safety and quality of care, while justice demands that patients are treated equitably, regardless of their participation in student education. Balancing educational needs with patient rights is essential to uphold ethical standards in healthcare.

**Substituted Judgment**
Substituted judgment is a principle in surrogate decision-making where a surrogate makes healthcare decisions based on what the patient would have chosen, rather than their own preferences. The surrogate must align their decisions with the patient's reasonable goals, values, and priorities, all within the boundaries of medical standards of care, institutional policies, and legal requirements. This is a positive right of the patient, ensuring their autonomy is respected even when they cannot make decisions themselves. When properly followed, substituted judgment is protected by a negative right, meaning others cannot interfere with the surrogate's decision.

**Surrogate Decision-Making**
Surrogate decision-making occurs when a designated individual makes healthcare decisions on behalf of a patient who is unable to do so. This practice is grounded in patient autonomy, with surrogates expected to use substituted judgment—making decisions based on what the patient would have chosen, aligned with their reasonable goals, values, and priorities. Ethical challenges arise when surrogates' beliefs conflict with the patient's preferences. Surrogates must act within medical standards, institutional policies, and legal mandates. Effective surrogate decision-making balances patient autonomy, beneficence, nonmaleficence, and justice, ensuring care that reflects the patient's best interests.

- *Cross-reference: Substituted Judgment, Advance Directive, Durable Power of Attorney (DPOA), Patient Autonomy*

# T

**Telemedicine**

Telemedicine leverages technology to deliver remote healthcare services, improving access for underserved and geographically isolated populations. While initially constrained by technology and cost, advancements have expanded its capabilities, offering real-time consultations and remote monitoring. However, telemedicine raises ethical dilemmas related to patient privacy, security, and the quality of care, particularly in the absence of physical exams. Federal regulations, such as HIPAA, ensure patient confidentiality, while telemedicine must align with patient autonomy, beneficence, nonmaleficence, and justice. Ensuring informed consent, safeguarding patient data, and addressing disparities in access are critical to ethically delivering telemedicine services.

**Terminal and Palliative Sedation**

Terminal or palliative sedation is used in end-of-life care to relieve intractable suffering by reducing a patient's consciousness without hastening death. Unlike euthanasia, its goal is to alleviate symptoms, not to shorten life. Ethical dilemmas arise regarding the balance between reducing suffering and the potential for life-shortening effects. Informed consent is crucial, ensuring patients or surrogates understand the permanent implications of sedation. Guided by the principles of autonomy, beneficence, nonmaleficence, and justice, terminal sedation is considered an ethically appropriate intervention when aligned with a patient's values and reasonable goals.

**Testimonials and Avoiding Quackery**

Testimonials have historically been used to promote unproven treatments, often leading to quackery, where claims are made without scientific validation. This practice raises significant ethical concerns about patient safety, informed consent, and the potential for misleading information. Modern ethical standards emphasize the need for transparency, requiring that testimonials used in healthcare be evidence-based and not mislead patients. Both the AMA and ACP stress the importance of promoting beneficence, nonmaleficence, and justice in healthcare marketing, ensuring that testimonials do not compromise patient autonomy or promote harmful, unproven therapies.

**Torture and Enhanced Interrogation**
Torture and enhanced interrogation involve coercive techniques, such as waterboarding and sleep deprivation, often used under the guise of extracting critical information, especially in military and political contexts. These practices have sparked global ethical, legal, and human rights debates, particularly regarding the balance between national security and human dignity. International law, including the United Nations Convention Against Torture (UNCAT), and U.S. legal protections like the Eighth Amendment, explicitly prohibit such methods. Ethical medical guidelines from organizations such as the AMA emphasize that healthcare professionals must not participate in or condone any form of torture or inhumane treatment.

**Triage Decision-Making**
Triage decision-making involves prioritizing patients based on the severity of their condition, particularly during emergencies when resources are limited. Originating in military medicine, triage aims to maximize survival by allocating care to those most likely to benefit. Contemporary dilemmas arise in balancing fairness, patient autonomy, and the ethical distribution of care, especially during crises like pandemics or disasters. Triage protocols must align with principles of beneficence, nonmaleficence, justice, and informed consent. Ensuring equitable access and transparency in decision-making is vital to maintaining trust in healthcare systems and upholding ethical standards.

# U

**Unemancipated Minor**

An unemancipated minor is an individual under the age of legal adulthood who has not been granted legal independence from their parents or guardians. In most jurisdictions, this means the minor is still under the care and control of their parents or guardians, who are responsible for making legal, medical, and financial decisions on their behalf. The rights and responsibilities of unemancipated minors vary by jurisdiction but generally include limitations on their ability to consent to medical treatments, enter into contracts, or make other significant legal decisions without parental or guardian approval

**Utilitarian Ethics**

Utilitarian ethics is a normative ethical theory that evaluates the moral worth of actions based on their outcomes or consequences. Founded by philosophers such as Jeremy Bentham and John Stuart Mill, this theory posits that the best action is the one that maximizes overall happiness or well-being and minimizes suffering. Utilitarianism advocates for making decisions that produce the greatest good for the greatest number of people. This consequentialist approach focuses on the results of actions rather than the intentions behind them or adherence to rules, emphasizing efficiency and overall impact in moral decision-making.

# V

**Virtue Ethics**

Virtue ethics is an ethical theory that emphasizes the role of character and virtue in moral decision-making, rather than focusing solely on the consequences of actions or adherence to rules. Rooted in the philosophy of Aristotle, virtue ethics asserts that moral behavior arises from cultivating virtuous traits such as courage, temperance, and wisdom. According to this theory, a virtuous person acts in ways that align with these moral virtues, leading to a flourishing and fulfilling life. Unlike deontological or consequentialist approaches, virtue ethics prioritizes the development of moral character and the intention behind actions, aiming for the enhancement of individual and communal well-being.

---

# W

**Weigh and Balance**

The Weigh and Balance process in ethical decision-making involves both the patient or surrogate and the practitioner collaboratively assessing the relative importance of the four primary bioethical principles: autonomy, beneficence, nonmaleficence, and justice. In the Weigh phase, they determine the weight of each principle based on the patient's reasonable goals, values, and priorities, while also considering medical standards of care, institutional policies, and legal mandates. In the Balance phase, they decide which principle or combination of principles should guide the decision-making process, aiming to arrive at a rational and reasonable recommendation that aligns with the patient's best interests and ethical obligations.

**Withholding and Withdrawing Treatment**

Withholding and withdrawing treatment refers to the ethical decision-making process of stopping or not initiating medical interventions when they no longer benefit the patient. Historically, medical ethics emphasized life preservation, but advancements in healthcare have raised dilemmas about when to forgo treatment that may prolong suffering. Contemporary practices prioritize patient autonomy, allowing individuals to refuse life-sustaining measures. Legal frameworks like the Patient Self-Determination Act (PSDA) support patient rights in these decisions. Balancing autonomy, beneficence, nonmaleficence, and justice ensures that care aligns with patients' values while preventing unnecessary harm.

---

# X

**Xenotransplantation**

Xenotransplantation refers to the transplantation of organs, tissues, or cells from one species to another, such as from animals to humans. This field raises significant ethical concerns, including issues of animal welfare, the potential for cross-species disease transmission, and the long-term implications for human health. Ethical debates focus on the justification for using animals in research and the possible impact on their well-being, as well as the need for rigorous safety testing and informed consent from patients who may receive xenotransplants. Additionally, considerations around the equitable distribution of such advanced treatments and their accessibility in different healthcare settings are central to the ethical discourse.

---

# Y

**Youth Consent**:

Youth consent involves the ethical and legal considerations surrounding the ability of minors to make informed decisions about their own medical care and treatment. In many jurisdictions, minors are considered legally unable to provide consent for certain medical procedures, requiring parental or guardian approval. However, exceptions exist for specific situations, such as emergency care or certain types of confidential services like reproductive health. The concept of the "mature minor doctrine" applies in some cases, allowing minors deemed mature enough to consent to their own care. Ethical issues include balancing the respect for adolescent autonomy with the need for parental involvement, ensuring that minors understand their medical choices, and protecting their rights to make decisions that impact their health and well-being.

- *Cross-reference: Informed Consent, Capacity, Minor Patients, Confidentiality.*

---

# Z

**Zoonotic Diseases and Public Health**

Zoonotic diseases, transmitted from animals to humans, have long impacted global health, with notable examples including the Black Death, rabies, and COVID-19. Historically, public health responses relied on quarantines and culling animals, raising ethical concerns about balancing human health, animal welfare, and environmental protection. Today, zoonotic diseases are exacerbated by urbanization and globalization, leading to ethical dilemmas regarding healthcare equity, resource allocation, and government mandates. Ethical responses to zoonotic outbreaks must balance autonomy, beneficence, nonmaleficence, and justice, ensuring fair and equitable access to healthcare while safeguarding public health.

- *Cross-reference: Public Health Ethics, Justice, Resource Allocation, Animal Welfare*

***

# Author

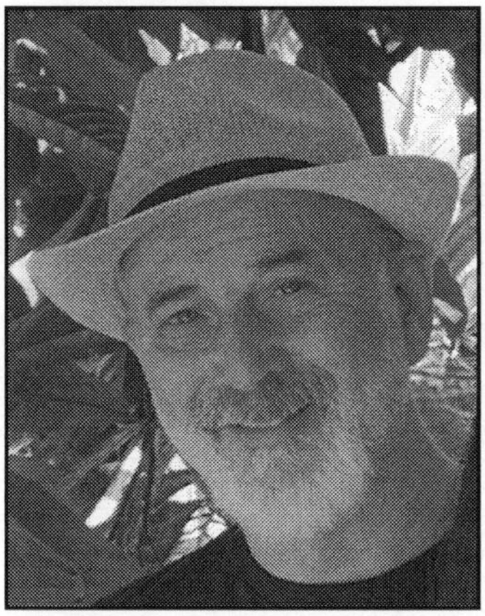

Dr. Jeffrey W. Bulger, PhD, has dedicated over 30 years to advancing bioethics consultation, policy development, and ethics education. He earned his PhD in Philosophy with a specialization in Medical Ethics from the University of Tennessee—Knoxville and was one of the first to be certified as a Healthcare Ethics Consultant (HEC-C). As Director of the Bioethics Program at The Chicago Medical School, Dr. Bulger has been instrumental in leading ethics consultations, developing ethical policies, and promoting ethics education within healthcare settings. His forthcoming book, *Bioethics: Passing the Boards, Providing Patient Care, and Beyond*, set to be published by Oxford University Press, reflects his continued dedication to integrating ethical principles into clinical practice.

In addition to his scholarly contributions, Dr. Bulger has chaired bioethics committees, mentored future leaders in the field, and advocated for the inclusion of bioethics in healthcare decision-making. He regularly engages in public and professional education, delivering presentations on a wide range of ethical topics. Dr. Bulger remains deeply committed to supporting the next generation of bioethics professionals, ensuring that ethical decision-making remains a cornerstone of patient care. His work continues to have a meaningful impact on shaping the ethical standards of healthcare today.

***

# Notes

# Notes

Made in the USA
Monee, IL
12 November 2026

834b8ca4-7f58-42b7-b6b1-f754fd15ac7cR01